UNDERSTANDING
HIGH-RISK PREGNANCY

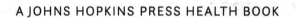

UNDERSTANDING HIGH-RISK PREGNANCY

A Patient's Guide to Prenatal Complications

ALAN M. PEACEMAN, MD

JOHNS HOPKINS UNIVERSITY PRESS
Baltimore

Note to the Reader: This book is not meant to substitute for medical care, and treatment should not be based solely on its contents. Instead, treatment must be developed in a dialogue between the individual and their physician. The book has been written to help with that dialogue. In view of ongoing research, changes in governmental regulation, and the constant flow of information relating to drug therapy and drug reactions, treatment recommendations may change subsequent to publication.

© 2025 Alan M. Peaceman
All rights reserved. Published 2025
Printed in the United States of America on acid-free paper
9 8 7 6 5 4 3 2 1

Johns Hopkins University Press
2715 North Charles Street
Baltimore, Maryland 21218
www.press.jhu.edu

Library of Congress Cataloging-in-Publication Data is available.

A catalog record for this book is available from the British Library.

ISBN 978-1-4214-5232-6 (hardcover)
ISBN 978-1-4214-5233-3 (paperback)
ISBN 978-1-4214-5234-0 (ebook)

Special discounts are available for bulk purchases of this book. For more information, please contact Special Sales at specialsales@jh.edu.

EU GPSR Authorized Representative
LOGOS EUROPE, 9 rue Nicolas Poussin, 17000, La Rochelle, France
E-mail: Contact@logoseurope.eu

To all of the women who put their trust
and that of their family in my care, and allowed me
to play a part in their pregnancy journey

CONTENTS

Preface ix

PART I BACKGROUND ON HIGH-RISK PREGNANCIES
1. High-Risk Pregnancy Basics *3*
2. Issues That Can Affect Pregnancy Outcomes *10*
3. Increased Risks in Black Women *20*

PART II EARLY PREGNANCY ISSUES
4. Preparing for Pregnancy and the First Trimester *27*
5. Miscarriage *34*

PART III MATERNAL CONDITIONS
6. Hypertension *43*
7. Diabetes *51*
8. Thyroid Disease *63*
9. Autoimmune Disorders: Lupus and Antiphospholipid Antibodies *68*
10. Heart Disease *78*
11. Kidney Disease *87*
12. Blood Clots: Pulmonary Embolism and Deep Vein Thrombosis *93*
13. Uterine Anomalies and Fibroids *99*
14. Cancer and Pregnancy *106*

PART IV **FETAL CONDITIONS**

15. Birth Defects *117*
16. Genetic Abnormalities *127*
17. Fetal Cardiac Arrhythmias *136*
18. Fetal Growth Restriction *143*
19. Congenital Infections *152*
20. Hydrops Fetalis *162*

PART V **PREGNANCY CONDITIONS**

21. Preterm Birth *171*
22. Preeclampsia *180*
23. Placental Abnormalities *190*
24. Stillbirth *203*
25. Blood Group Isoimmunization *211*
26. Cervical Insufficiency *220*
27. Multiple Gestation *226*

Conclusion 234
Glossary 239
Notes 247
Index 259

PREFACE

Pregnancy can be a wonderful time in a woman's life. There is the anticipation of bringing a new life into the world, the thrill of feeling this new being moving inside of you, the bond that grows as the pregnancy progresses, and the dreams that come with the future of family life. Pregnancy is a natural process, but also can rightly bring a sense of accomplishment and pride in the power of the female body.

However, not all pregnancies are straightforward and routine. Many women have conditions or factors that add a degree of difficulty and risk of complications. And the number of pregnancies that are threatened by high-risk conditions has increased significantly over the past few decades. These complications can lead to more office visits, more recommended testing, and possibly hospitalization, early delivery, or even pregnancy loss.

This book, which is meant to be helpful to the average patient like yourself, will not focus on issues related to routine pregnancy. Instead, it will describe many high-risk conditions—some that affect women before they become pregnant, others that arise during pregnancy—that can complicate pregnancy and explain how they are diagnosed and treated. The book offers the same counsel I've given to thousands of patients with these issues during my many years of practice. I have loved helping patients through complicated pregnancies and celebrating with them when their dreams of a healthy child have come true. I have enjoyed educating them about their condition and sharing their relief when I can reassure them that the prognosis is good. Being a maternal-fetal medicine specialist has been a very rewarding career, and I am glad to be able to share my expertise with a wider audience.

My goal in writing this book is to help you better understand your situation and to answer questions you may already have. It may also help guide you in discussions with your medical provider. In many instances, it will provide reassurance and relieve some of your anxiety; at other times it may raise concerns you may not have considered. As a physician who has practiced high-risk obstetrics for over 30 years, I've always explained to my patients not just what should be done, but also why. The book examines the most common issues and complications encountered in today's high-risk obstetric practice. After reading it, I hope you will understand more about your pregnancy and how it can be managed and monitored. This knowledge will make you more comfortable with the risks involved and create reasonable expectations for the possible outcomes.

The book is divided into several sections. Part I gives you some background on high-risk pregnancies and external factors that can affect pregnancy, including environmental influences and mental health. In part II, I discuss conception and early pregnancy issues, including miscarriage. I also examine issues related to the age of the mother. Part III is about medical conditions that women may already have, such as diabetes, hypertension, and immune disorders, and how these could affect the pregnancy. Part IV includes chapters about fetal conditions that may be identified during pregnancy, including birth defects and infections. Part V describes preeclampsia, multiple gestation, preterm birth, as well as other obstetric complications that do not fit into the other categories. Many of the conditions covered also feature patients' case studies to provide a more intimate view of what you might expect during pregnancy when dealing with the same situation. Their names have been changed to protect their privacy.

You are likely reading this book because your doctor told you that you are high risk. "High risk" is a broad and generic term that covers a multitude of conditions and health concerns. Up to 30% of pregnant women have risk factors for complications, but many of these are minor and do not need any special treatment. Others are of more concern and require some modification of care but are still likely to result in a good outcome and a healthy baby. Some conditions, however, are very serious and have the potential for life-threatening complications for the mother or the baby. This book contains examples of all these risk factors. Some women have more than one of these complications, but no one gets them all. Just remember that with all of the advances in diagnostics and emerging technologies, women are now in a better place than ever before to bring their pregnancies to term and deliver healthy babies.

When faced with a medical problem, many patients are immediately frightened and have difficulty absorbing the information shared with them. I intend to present each condition clearly and hope to reduce this fear so that you can then learn about your situation and understand how best to deal with it. My experience is that a discussion which includes background on the condition, what the risks are, how it is monitored, and approaches to treatment can be beneficial for reducing fear and anxiety, increasing communication and trust between the physician and patient, and improving outcomes. If this book can accomplish any of these goals, I believe you will find it worthwhile. I wish you the best on your journey through pregnancy.

UNDERSTANDING
HIGH-RISK PREGNANCY

PART I

BACKGROUND ON HIGH-RISK PREGNANCIES

CHAPTER 1

HIGH-RISK PREGNANCY BASICS

THERE ARE BETWEEN three and four million births in the United States every year, making it one of the most common medical conditions that American women experience. For first-time mothers in particular, it can be a time of joyful anticipation as they watch their bodies grow and change to create new life. Most of these pregnancies are uncomplicated and result in healthy outcomes for the mother and her baby. These routine pregnancies are a natural experience and can give the newborn a healthy start to childhood. However, up to 30% of pregnant women have high-risk issues, which can affect their maternal health, the outcome of the pregnancy, and the care they receive. If you are one of these women, understanding your issues and getting the appropriate care for them can contribute not only to a better outcome but also reduce anxiety and worry that can detract from the pregnancy experience.

WHAT IS A HIGH-RISK PREGNANCY?

You may find it strange that there is no single accepted definition of what constitutes a high-risk pregnancy. Probably more than half of women will have at least one risk factor that could be an issue, but for most of these women it will minimally affect their pregnancy care or the outcome. For other women, their risk factor could seriously impact their health or the health of the baby. The focus should be on those risk factors and complications that can affect pregnancy outcomes, and how they are managed.

WHO MANAGES PREGNANCIES WITH RISK FACTORS AND COMPLICATIONS?

Becoming a physician who cares for women during pregnancy requires many years of training. After college and medical school, a physician who desires to focus on the care of women and pregnancy will do a residency in obstetrics and gynecology. This is a four-year program of education and hands-on experience during which the physician receives training in routine gynecologic care, pregnancy and delivery management, infertility, and gynecologic cancers. At the conclusion of this residency, the physician is then eligible to become board certified in obstetrics and gynecology and can practice independently. Board certification is granted by the American Board of Obstetrics and Gynecology (ABOG) after the physician successfully completes both written and oral examinations. These practitioners are referred to as obstetrics and gynecology generalists, and on occasion as obstetric generalists. Nurse midwives and family medicine physicians can also provide pregnancy care and do deliveries, but these practitioners primarily manage pregnant patients without significant risk factors.

Some physicians choose to perform further subspecialty training in management of pregnancy complications through a fellowship in maternal-fetal medicine (MFM). This additional three years of education and training focuses on managing pregnancy risk factors and more serious complications. Upon completing this fellowship, the physician is eligible to become additionally certified in the subspecialty of maternal-fetal medicine. This additional certification requires successful completion of both written and oral examinations administered by ABOG which are more focused on pregnancy complications.

Not all pregnancy risk factors require evaluation and care by an MFM subspecialist. Many are within the scope of expertise of obstetric generalists. On occasion a general obstetrician or a midwife will refer a patient to an MFM subspecialist for a consultation to assess the level of risk and create a plan of care, and the patient will then return to the referring provider for her ongoing prenatal care and delivery. Some MFM physicians only provide this type of consultative care and do not perform deliveries, while other MFM practices care for the patient during the entire pregnancy and postdelivery (postpartum) period.

Knowing the distinctions between these areas of maternal care can help you make a more informed decision about the medical professional you choose and entrust your care to during your pregnancy.

GESTATIONAL AGE

Although a pregnancy's due date is at 40 weeks' gestation, all pregnancies are considered to be full term at 37 weeks. Nevertheless, there is still a benefit to the fetus for going further. At 37–38 weeks, 8.2% of babies are admitted to the neonatal ICU (NICU), mostly for some mild issues related to immaturity. At 39–40 weeks, 6.2% have NICU admission, and at 41 or more weeks the percentage of babies admitted to the NICU is 7.8%.[1] There is other evidence that going past 39 weeks may not be of benefit. When low-risk women in their first pregnancy were randomized to induction at 39 weeks versus waiting at least until 41 weeks for labor to start, the induction group had 16% fewer cesarean deliveries, 20% fewer neonatal complications, and 10% fewer NICU admissions.[2] For twin gestations the average gestational age at delivery is 36 weeks, and

32 weeks for triplets.[3] Most babies born at 32 weeks or after have few complications in the nursery, and with modern technology and health care interventions, babies born prior to this point can often survive with no long-term disabilities. (Complications of prematurity will be discussed further in chapter 21.)

MEDICATION USE DURING PREGNANCY

It is common knowledge that the use of certain medications can have adverse effects on a pregnancy. The most well-known instance of this is thalidomide used in the 1950s and 1960s to treat morning sickness, which tragically caused severe limb deformities in some babies born to mothers who used it. Another example was the decades-long use of DES, a form of estrogen intended to prevent miscarriages. DES was linked to uterine birth defects and vaginal cancer years later in some women born to mothers who took it. Physicians have learned from these examples and are now more cautious about prescribing medication to pregnant women. However, it is much easier to show that a drug causes harm than to prove with certainty that a medication is safe to take during pregnancy. Many drugs have been given to pregnant women for years without being linked to birth defects, and these are *presumed* to be safe. Examples of these are insulin and thyroid hormones. A few medications are associated with a very high risk of birth defects, such as retinoic acid (also known as Accutane), a derivative of vitamin A used for treating acne. There are medications associated with a lower risk (less than 3%) of causing birth defects which are still avoided if possible, such as certain anti-seizure medications. And then there is the largest group of medications where there is some level of uncertainty.

You and your provider should discuss medications you are currently taking, as well as those being prescribed during pregnancy so you can weigh the benefits versus the risks. Every obstetric provider discusses common medications multiple times every day, so don't shy away from asking. In some instances, a physician will still recommend a medication that has some known risk, but this is usually a situation where this is the best or only medication to treat the mother's serious health condition and the risk of the medication causing an adverse effect on the fetus is relatively low. Examples of this might be warfarin (a blood thinner) for patients with a mechanical heart valve, and chemotherapy to treat cancer. But the most common situation is where there is significant experience over many years with use of a medication during pregnancy with no apparent increase in adverse effects on the fetus. Even without randomized controlled trials that *prove* that they are safe, these medications are presumed to be acceptable for use in pregnancy as long as there is an appropriate indication. The list of these medications presumed to be safe include acetaminophen (Tylenol) and many cold remedies, but also many drugs used to treat other medical conditions. The discussion will often come down to the benefits of the medicines far outweighing any theoretical but unseen risks that might remain, and you should feel comfortable taking them.

One of the many changes to your body during pregnancy is an increase in the amount of circulating blood. Maternal blood volume can increase 50% by the third trimester compared with pre-pregnancy, and even more in twin pregnancies. This increased blood volume delivers the extra nutrients and oxygen required by the developing fetus, and it allows the mother to tolerate the normal bleeding that occurs during and after delivery. With this increased blood volume, doses of medication may need to be adjusted as pregnancy advances to maintain a steady blood level.

With more attention to mental health today, more women of reproductive age are being treated with medications for depression and anxiety. Concerns have been raised with a few of these drugs when taken during pregnancy, but for most medications the concerns have not been consistent or conclusive. Some women will choose to stop their medication during pregnancy, while others feel it is vital to their ability to function. If you currently take medication for any mental health issue, ensure your care provider addresses your needs and supports the continuation of your medications if warranted.

Concern about the development of postpartum depression (PPD) is also appropriate. Patients with a history of depression or an anxiety disorder are known to be at increased risk for developing PPD. Sertraline (Zoloft) is a medication used for depression and anxiety disorders that many physicians are most comfortable with during pregnancy and breastfeeding—it has a track record of use now for many years and by thousands of patients without evidence of adverse effects. Even for patients not on it during pregnancy, it may be recommended that medication be started during pregnancy if depression symptoms warrant it. It may also be reasonable to start it a month or so before anticipated delivery for those at risk of PPD, as it often takes a few weeks to see beneficial effects.

ULTRASOUND

The introduction of ultrasound examinations into routine clinical practice in the 1980s revolutionized obstetric care. The field of obstetrics transformed from caring for one patient (only the mother) to caring for two. Before routine ultrasound use, birth defects were rarely identified before birth, and the presence of twins was frequently unknown until delivery. In the United States and many other countries today, almost all women have at least one ultrasound during pregnancy, and most have more than one.

Ultrasound can assess fetal structure and function—it can identify organs that do not appear to have developed normally and those not doing what they are supposed to do. It can see a heart which is not pumping blood very well, an abnormal growth of tissue in the lungs, kidneys that are not making urine, legs that are not moving, and growth that is lagging.

Ultrasound is an amazing tool that continues to improve with advances in technology. All evidence suggests that it is safe to use and does not harm the fetus, but it should only be used when there is a medical indication. For the high-risk conditions described in this book, ultrasound can be an essential tool in pregnancy management, and can be used as often as needed without concerns for adverse effects.

These are some basic issues that are relevant to high-risk pregnancies. We will cover others in the chapters to come. In chapter 2, we will cover issues that can cause a pregnancy to be high risk.

CHAPTER 2

ISSUES THAT CAN AFFECT PREGNANCY OUTCOMES

MANY NONMEDICAL FACTORS can influence the outcome of any pregnancy, causing a high-risk situation where none might have been present. While some can be modified, most cannot. Most women are aware that both smoking and alcohol use during pregnancy have adverse effects on the developing fetus, and many women can reduce or eliminate their use. Illicit drug use is always discouraged as well. And being Black is now recognized as associated with higher rates of maternal mortality. But there are other less discussed issues that have the potential for adversely impacting the outcome of a pregnancy. This chapter explores many of these issues that could affect your pregnancy.

SMOKING DURING PREGNANCY

Every pack of cigarettes now sold in the United States has a health warning label printed on it. There are 11 different warnings which can appear, one of which concerns smoking during pregnancy. "Smoking during pregnancy stunts fetal growth" is printed on some cigarette packs, along with a picture of a baby on a scale weighing four pounds. Previously, some packaging carried the label, "SURGEON

GENERAL'S WARNING: Smoking By Pregnant Women May Result in Fetal Injury, Premature Birth, And Low Birth Weight." It should be clear to everyone who smokes that smoking is bad for your health, and results in more pregnancy complications.

The prevalence of smoking in the United States has dropped significantly since the first surgeon general's report in 1964. Yet almost one in eight American adults continues to smoke, according to the Centers for Disease Control and Prevention (CDC),[1] with rates higher in many other countries. The rate in 2021 was highest for those age 25–44 at 12.6%. Although the percentage of mothers who smoked cigarettes at any time during pregnancy declined by 36% from 2016 to 2021, almost 5% of pregnant women still smoke.[2]

The list of obstetric complications linked to tobacco use is extensive. It includes delay in getting pregnant, miscarriage, birth defects, fetal growth restriction, premature birth, damage to the baby's developing lungs and brain, placental abruption, stillbirth, and sudden infant death syndrome (SIDS). For those with nicotine dependence, quitting smoking is difficult, but the health benefits during pregnancy are worth the struggle. Many programs exist to assist patients with this, and you can find access to them on the internet or from your health care provider. If smoking cessation cannot be achieved, nicotine replacement therapy, often in the form of a nicotine patch but available in gum or other forms, should be considered, as the general consensus is that using other forms of nicotine is better than smoking.

ALCOHOL USE IN PREGNANCY

As with cigarettes there has been extensive public education about the concerns of alcohol use during pregnancy. Since 1988, all alcoholic beverages sold in the United States must carry the following warning: "GOVERNMENT WARNING: According to the Surgeon General, women should not drink alcoholic beverages during pregnancy because of the risk of birth defects." Fetal alcohol syndrome disorders (FASD) are often characterized by some facial features (small eyes, thin upper lip, and a smooth skin surface between the nose and mouth) which often go unrecognized. More importantly, FASD can cause slowed growth of the fetus before birth, and then behavioral abnormalities, which can include lack of coordination, poor fine-motor skills, learning disabilities, hyperactivity, and attention deficit. FASD is more common with increasing amounts of alcohol consumption, but no amount of alcohol is known to be safe.[3] Binge drinking is thought to be more of a risk than low levels of alcohol consumption, but even lower levels of drinking raise concerns. The general recommendation is therefore to abstain from drinking any alcohol during pregnancy.

Total abstention from alcohol use in pregnancy is good advice, but it may cause fear, anxiety, and regret among women who consumed a glass of wine or a cocktail prior to recognizing that they were pregnant or during the course of their pregnancies. Many women are concerned that they might have caused permanent brain injury to their unborn child by having had one or two alcoholic drinks. It is reassuring that the scientific literature does not show a link between very light alcohol consumption during early pregnancy and FASD.[4] There is no evidence that it is 100% safe, either, so abstinence should be encouraged. But consuming a small amount of alcohol early in pregnancy should not be a major source of worry.

OPIOID-USE DISORDER (OUD)

Opioid abuse has a long history going back centuries, but only recently has it reached crisis proportions in the United States. Opiates are naturally occurring compounds derived from the poppy plant, while the term "opioids" refers to both natural opiates and laboratory-synthesized compounds. Opioid-use disorder (OUD) can be defined as a chronic brain disease where there is a craving or urge to use opioids and development of tolerance, with unsuccessful efforts to control this use, causing interference with social function and dangerous behavior. Opioid use can lead to viral infections including HIV and hepatitis C from sharing needles, nutritional deficiencies, emergency room visits, an irregular heart rate, and death. Annual opioid overdose deaths in the United States have risen dramatically from approximately 8,400 in 2000 to 47,600 in 2017, to over 80,000 in 2021.[5] Over 2 million Americans meet criteria for a past-year OUD.[6]

Opioids per se are not harmful during pregnancy for the mother or the fetus. They can be prescribed for severe pain which can occasionally occur due to surgery, trauma, and other uncommon situations. Chronic opioid use, however, can be a significant concern. It has been linked to poor fetal growth, preterm birth, stillbirth, and the neonatal abstinence syndrome (NAS).[7] NAS is opioid withdrawal in the newborn, and can be characterized by trembling, irritability, poor sleep, seizures, and poor feeding. It usually requires prolonged hospitalization of the newborn until symptoms subside and appropriate feeding and growth is established.

The American College of Obstetricians and Gynecologists (ACOG) now recommends screening all pregnant women for substance use at the first prenatal visit. If identified, referral for treatment can improve maternal and infant outcomes.[8] Treatment of OUD during pregnancy can be difficult; quick withdrawal for opioid dependence is not recommended, as it can lead to miscarriage or preterm labor. Use of medications is commonly recommended over supervised withdrawal, as it is associated with a lower risk of relapse. Medications including methadone and buprenorphine are both options, but buprenorphine is becoming the preferred drug. It can be prescribed by any physicians who complete the training, comes in the form of a pill, has a lower risk of overdose and fewer side effects than methadone, and is associated with a lower risk of NAS.

ENVIRONMENT

A number of studies have examined the impact of exposure to environmental contaminants on the developing fetus. Maternal smoking effects were described above, but maternal exposure to secondhand smoke has also been linked to respiratory disorders in the developing fetus.[9] Air pollution has also been linked to complications in the fetus, including low birth weight, preterm birth, and abnormal lung function.[10,11] There is a wide variety of environmental toxins and hormones which raise concerns about their effects on the developing fetus, including mercury in fish, lead in the drinking water, pesticides in the food supply, heavy metal exposure in some workplaces, estrogenic chemicals in plastics, and microplastics found nearly everywhere. In today's society, it is impossible to avoid most of these exposures, and their individual effects are difficult to tease out. The impact is probably worst in low socioeconomic areas, where pollution levels are often the highest. The ACOG advice to reduce the risks associated with these pollutants includes cleaning with nontoxic products, avoiding using pesticides at home, eating fish with lower levels of mercury, washing all raw produce, even if it will be peeled, and choosing nonplastic containers for food and drink.[12]

IVF PREGNANCIES

In vitro fertilization (IVF) is an amazing procedure which has brought families to countless infertile couples over the past 40 years. Women of any age with difficulty conceiving or with partners with fertility challenges, as well as women in menopause, are now able to have pregnancies through IVF with their own or donor eggs. Success rates have improved dramatically so that single embryo transfer is now common. Along with these successes, however, comes the caveat that IVF pregnancies have a higher risk of complications than do naturally conceived pregnancies. Multiple gestations are still more common in IVF pregnancies, along with their associated risks (chapter 27). In addition, women who have IVF pregnancies are more likely to develop hypertension, gestational diabetes, placenta previa, and placental abruption, and are more likely to be delivered by cesarean.[13] Fetal congenital heart defects are also more common in IVF pregnancies. As such, IVF pregnancies require more monitoring for complications than do naturally conceived pregnancies. Some medications used to treat infertility also increase the risk of having a multiple gestation, but not the other risks associated with IVF.

MENTAL HEALTH

Pregnant women, like everyone, often say that they are, to varying degrees, "stressed." Many women express concern that their level of stress will adversely impact their pregnancy, and some data regarding preterm birth support this concern. But it is very difficult to quantify the contribution of stress to adverse outcomes. Eliminating stress from one's life is not a realistic goal, but stress reduction—which may be achieved through yoga, meditation, or exercise, as examples—is probably good for everyone. So consider ways that you may be able to limit excessive responsibilities and find time for relaxation. You are likely familiar with stress-reducing activities like meditation, walking in nature, talking to a friend, getting good sleep, keeping social contacts, and journaling.

When a pregnancy starts off in the high-risk category, as it does, say, for twin pregnancies, stress levels can be increased. This stress of a high-risk pregnancy can be quite disturbing and can interfere with your ability to function on a day-to-day basis. It can be even more difficult for women with a history of an adverse outcome in a prior pregnancy. Counseling with a professional who has experience helping women with difficult pregnancies can be very helpful. As already discussed in chapter 1, antidepression medication may be appropriate and help you deal with the stress.

There are other mental health conditions that can affect women during pregnancy, including chronic anxiety/depression and bipolar disorder. In fact, one in four pregnant women meet the criteria for an anxiety disorder.[14] Women with these conditions are often on medication prior to pregnancy to help control them. Stopping these medications when you find out that you are pregnant is never a good idea without talking with the provider who is monitoring your condition. Sudden discontinuation of some medications can trigger worse symptoms. Some medications are thought to be safe and should be continued during pregnancy. At times, transition to a different medication will be recommended. Untreated psychiatric disorders can interfere with day-to-day function, and can be a risk to the mother as well as the fetus. Treatment of mental health conditions is an important part of medical care and should be addressed appropriately like any other medical condition.

MATERNAL AGE

If you are 35 or older and either pregnant or thinking about having a baby, you are not alone. The average age for women having babies in this country and around the developed world has increased significantly over the past two decades, and the percentage of women having children after age 35 has increased as well. The teenage pregnancy rate in the United States has dropped dramatically, and the percentage of births to women over 35 has increased 40% since 2000 (table 2.1). Even births to women in their forties and fifties has been increasing, often with the assistance of fertility treatments. Presumably this increase in maternal age is related to more women entering the work force and having careers, as well as more consistent use of effective birth control methods. Yet pregnancy after age

Table 2.1 Percentage of Births by Maternal Age

	2000	2005	2010	2015	2020
<20	11.8%	10.2%	9.3%	5.8%	4.4%
20-24	25.1%	25.1%	23.8%	21.4%	18.4%
25-29	26.8%	27.3%	28.3%	29.0%	28.3%
30-34	22.9%	23.0%	24.1%	27.5%	29.6%
35-39	11.1%	11.7%	11.6%	13.3%	15.6%
>39	2.3%	2.7%	2.9%	3.0%	3.6%

Source: Centers for Disease Control and Prevention, National Center for Health Statistics. National Vital Statistics System, Natality on CDC WONDER Online Database. Data are from the Natality Records 2007–2022, as compiled from data provided by the 57 vital statistics jurisdictions through the Vital Statistics Cooperative Program. Accessed at http://wonder.cdc.gov/natality-current.html

35 has been thought to be riskier, and sometimes referred to as advanced maternal age.

Studies have long shown that pregnancy in older women is associated with increased risks of complications for both the mother and the fetus. Mothers have a higher incidence of developing preeclampsia, gestational diabetes, and miscarriage, and rates of cesarean are also increased. It is not surprising that as we get older, we are more likely to have acquired a diagnosis of a chronic condition, such as diabetes or hypertension, than when we were in our twenties. Being overweight or obese is also more common with aging. These conditions are a major reason why pregnancy complications are more common among women over 35. One study found that compared to women in their twenties, the severe complication rate for women aged 35–39 was 40% higher, for women aged 40–44 was almost double, and for women 45 and older it was more than triple.[15] For the fetus born of a woman over 35, there are higher rates of preterm birth, growth restriction, and stillbirth, primarily after age 40. Some fetal complications are related to underlying maternal conditions, but the increase in complications is also seen in healthy women. Rates of chromosomal abnormalities, such as Down syndrome, also increase with maternal age. Women over the age of 35 at the time of delivery should be aware of these concerns. Nonetheless, you need to remember that although these risks are elevated relative to younger mothers, most women aged 35 and older are still able to have healthy babies without major complications.

MANAGEMENT OF PREGNANCY AT AGE 35 AND OLDER

The pregnancy care for women aged 35 and above is not too different from the care provided for younger women. If a chronic condition or illness is present, the recommendations are as outlined for that condition later in this book. For women without an underlying condition, the options for genetic testing should be made available, as described in chapter 4. To reduce the risk of preeclampsia, a single, daily, low-dose aspirin tablet is recommended beginning between 12–16 weeks until delivery. Ultrasounds should be performed to look for birth defects and to assess fetal growth. And due to the higher rate of stillbirth at age 40 and after, initiating weekly fetal surveillance in the third trimester with either a nonstress test (NST) or biophysical profile (BPP, both explained in chapter 6), and proceeding with delivery by the mother's due date is frequently recommended.

While it should be recognized that some of the risks of pregnancy are increased with advancing maternal age, you should also recognize that the odds of a successful pregnancy outcome are still very much in your favor. Most women who are in good health entering pregnancy, and those with an underlying medical condition which is well controlled, have a favorable prognosis. With the appropriate care and some extra testing, women beyond the age of 35 are most likely going to have a healthy child without a major risk to their own health.

SUMMARY

Both medical and nonmedical factors can influence the outcome of pregnancy, sending it from a low-risk category to a high-risk one. You should be aware of these factors, and limit your exposure as much as possible. You are encouraged to discuss these issues with your provider whenever they arise and seek assistance from other sources that are available. Doing so may not only increase the chances of having a better outcome for you and your baby but also reduce your level of anxiety.

CHAPTER 3

INCREASED RISKS IN BLACK WOMEN

SADLY, RACIAL DIFFERENCES continue to impact maternal health and pregnancy outcomes, with little progress being made in leveling the playing field. Black women have twice the rate of preterm birth as their White or Hispanic counterparts, even after controlling for socioeconomic status. Babies of Black women are also twice as likely to die before or soon after birth than babies of White women.[1] And appropriately, there is continuing media attention on the more than double rate of maternal mortality for Black women despite efforts to address this issue. American Indian and Alaska Native women also have much higher rates of these complications. The reasons for these differences are multifactorial, with preexisting conditions, environment, implicit and explicit bias, psychosocial stress, access to care, and genetics all likely playing a part. Progress in correcting these inequalities has been very slow but could have a major impact on racial differences in outcomes. Until then, it is all the more important for Black women to understand conditions that contribute to high-risk pregnancies and the treatment options available to ensure that they receive the care that they deserve.

PREEXISTING CONDITIONS

Much of the difference in maternal mortality rates between races is due to two complications—hypertension and thrombosis (blood clots). Both of these conditions lead to death more frequently in the Black population, as does diabetes, hemorrhage during delivery, and heart disease.[2] Black women can educate themselves about their risks of these conditions and how best to reduce these risks, and then they should make sure their provider takes these risks into account. Attention to these conditions will be important for efforts to reduce the disproportionately high rates of maternal morbidity and mortality in Black women. Management of these conditions should be similar for all women, and will be discussed in chapters that follow.

ENVIRONMENT

As discussed in chapter 2, environment can play an important role in pregnancy complications and newborn development. People of lower socioeconomic status are more likely to live in areas with high levels of air pollution and other chemical toxins. They are also more likely to live in areas with less access to healthy food choices, and diet quality not only affects nutrient intake but also obesity rates. Obesity is a major contributor to rates of diabetes and hypertension and also increases the risk of birth defects and stillbirth. Personal safety can also be an environmental issue, with homicides accounting for almost 10% of maternal deaths. These environmental issues affect Black Americans more than White Americans. Until the inequities in these risk factors are corrected, the environment will continue to be a contributor to disparities in obstetric outcomes.

IMPLICIT AND EXPLICIT BIAS

Patients depend on receiving high-quality care from their providers, and high-quality care depends on communication. Good communication between the patient and her provider will generate mutual respect and diminish patient fear and distrust, and will facilitate information gathering, accurate diagnosis, appropriate counseling, shared decision-making, better patient compliance with recommendations, and realistic expectations. Language differences can be a barrier to good communication, as can lack of understanding of the patient's culture and social situation. Poor communication can be due to poor provider skills, provider time constraints, and patient resistance. But it can also be due to provider biases.

With explicit bias, an individual is aware of prejudices and attitudes toward certain groups, while with implicit bias the individual is not consciously aware of this prejudice. Both types of bias can affect communication and decision-making, negatively impacting the patient. In particular, Black women have reported their concerns not being taken seriously, being talked down to, being blamed for adverse outcomes, and in general being stereotyped.[3] They believe that this leads to substandard medical care and less attention to their pain. This issue is exacerbated by the relatively low numbers of women of color in the obstetric care community. It is easy to see how bias can lead to differences in outcomes between races. But how much this contributes to the disparity in outcomes is not measurable. If you feel as though your health care team is not listening or attending to your concerns or symptoms, it is okay to press for better responses, or to switch doctors if that is warranted. It is always appropriate to advocate on your own behalf.

PSYCHOSOCIAL STRESS

There is a body of literature that links both acute and chronic stress during pregnancy with both preterm birth and low birth weight. Biomedical and psychosocial stressors can affect the neuroendocrine system, which can in turn trigger adaptive responses in different organs, which can negatively impact the pregnancy. Shorter pregnancy intervals were measured when women in the first trimester experienced the Northridge earthquake in California in 1994 and were near the World Trade Center on September 11, 2001.[4] Chronic stress not associated with a single event but assessed through composite measures of perceived stress have also been associated with preterm birth. In one study, women with high levels of anxiety and those who perceive having experienced racial discrimination had double the risk of preterm delivery.[5]

Biomarkers have been identified to measure the cumulative effects of exposure to stress over one's lifetime, and abnormal measures have been correlated with preterm birth, low birth weight, and preeclampsia. And Black women have the highest measures of these biomarkers.[6]

ACCESS TO CARE

There are many socioeconomic factors which can affect access to quality health care. Financial constraints and lack of health insurance can be barriers to prenatal appointments, medications, and recommended testing. Distance from a care center and inadequate public transportation can make keeping appointments difficult. Childcare issues, inability to miss work for appointments, and unstable housing can also be factors. Insufficient numbers of providers willing to serve the disadvantaged community may limit the services available. And prior bad experiences with the health care community may disincline women from seeking timely care.[7]

All of these factors can contribute to nonrecognition and assessment of high risk factors, late presentation with pregnancy complications, and overall worse outcomes for the mother and child.

GENETICS

Genetics plays an important role in susceptibility to disease. Patients from different racial and ethnic backgrounds have differing frequencies of some genes that have been associated with cancer, genetic disorders, and diabetes, among other conditions. It is likely that genetic differences between Black Americans and White Americans plays some role in disparities in pregnancy outcomes as well. Some genes associated with either preeclampsia or preterm birth are more common in Black Americans. How much these genetic differences contribute to overall disparities is uncertain and difficult to quantitate. The social issues described above likely contribute much more.

SUMMARY

As you can see, there are many issues that can affect pregnancy outcomes for Black women other than the better-known high-risk factors. While some are person specific, others are environmental or social. The medical community has recognized the disparities in outcomes, especially with regard to maternal mortality, and has begun taking steps to address the inequality. These steps include increased funding for research into the causes of disparities, mandated training in diversity and forms of bias, and increasing the diversity in medical school admissions and medical leadership. Changes in the societal contribution to disparate outcomes is likely to occur more slowly.

PART II

EARLY PREGNANCY ISSUES

CHAPTER 4

PREPARING FOR PREGNANCY AND THE FIRST TRIMESTER

IN AN IDEAL WORLD, all pregnancies would be planned and desired. Before deciding to start a family, couples would use birth control methods, and these would never fail to prevent an unplanned pregnancy. Women would be in their best state of health, and any medical conditions that they have would be optimally controlled. The risks of pregnancy would be recognized and accepted. In reality, however, for many women or couples, pregnancy occurs without conditions being ideal. No birth control method short of sterilization or total abstinence is 100% effective, nor is it utilized with every episode of intercourse. When a woman becomes pregnant, she may not yet have quit smoking or drinking alcohol. She may be taking medication and unsure if it is appropriate for use during pregnancy. She may also be worried about her weight. Any of these situations can lead to concerns and worry.

It is important for all women to receive gynecologic care as a routine part of their primary care. This should include the provision of birth control if desired until they are ready to conceive, and a discussion about pregnancy beforehand. Your discussion with your gynecologist is an opportunity to ask questions about preparing for pregnancy and any changes you should make. If you have a specialist you see for a medical complication, it would be important to discuss pregnancy plans with this provider as well. Recommendations may be made to delay pregnancy until specific tests are completed or an underlying condition is better controlled. Medications may be altered to ones considered safer for pregnancy. It may also be recommended that you meet with a maternal-fetal medicine specialist in consultation before conception to discuss the risks and prognosis for pregnancy and make plans for your medical care during the prenatal period, especially if you have some specific health concerns.

Today, anyone can take a home pregnancy test soon after a missed period. Home pregnancy tests are very accurate and can demonstrate a positive result two weeks after conception occurs. In most cases, it is not necessary to visit your doctor until at least four to six weeks after conception. During that visit, you will likely get an ultrasound to confirm that the pregnancy is in the uterus, not ectopic (forming in the fallopian tubes). The ultrasound will also look for any signs of a developing miscarriage, and help to establish the due date. Before the first visit, if you have not previously discussed the medications you are currently taking, you may want to contact your provider for instructions.

The main concern before this time would be if you develop persistent lower abdominal pain, which could indicate an ectopic pregnancy—when the embryo gets stuck in the fallopian tube rather than developing in the uterus. This is a very dangerous situation because the tube could rupture, leading to internal hemorrhage. If you are experiencing this type of pain, you should contact your doctor right away.

THE FIRST PRENATAL VISIT

At the first prenatal visit, it is important to establish how far along the pregnancy is. This information is critical if you are considered high risk, since many important decisions depend on knowing how far along you are in the pregnancy. Some women will know the exact date of conception, but more often conception is estimated to have occurred in the middle of the woman's cycle. Using the first day of the last menstrual period (LMP) to determine the due date is often imprecise, as cycles vary in length and regularity, but that is often how due dates are determined. When fertility treatments are used for conception, there can be precise dating. Otherwise, it is often helpful to measure the size of the embryo (the developing fetus before eight weeks after conception) using ultrasound at the first prenatal visit to determine if it correlates with the size expected with dating from the first day of the LMP. If it correlates, the due date is then exactly 40 completed weeks after the LMP. You may think it is odd that you are already at two weeks of gestation when conception occurs, but this is how it is counted. It will then be 38 weeks from conception until the estimated due date, which is roughly nine months.

A medical history and physical examination are routinely done at a first prenatal visit, and laboratory testing is ordered. Routine laboratory tests will include tests for blood type, red blood count to check for anemia, hepatitis B, and syphilis. Other tests may be ordered based on other risk factors you might have. You should discuss options for genetic testing, and a plan for the ongoing care, including frequency of visits and future tests to be performed. This is also the time when risk factors are discussed—what their implications may be for your pregnancy and how it will affect your care management. The first visit offers an important opportunity for you to ask questions and know the plan for going forward (see box 4.1).

GENETIC TESTING

Humans have 23 pairs of chromosomes, each containing thousands of genes. Having an extra chromosome or missing one—or missing

> **BOX 4.1   COMPONENTS OF THE FIRST PRENATAL VISIT**
>
> - Establishing pregnancy dating
> - Medical history and physical examination
> - Options for genetic testing
> - Ultrasound
> - Laboratory tests
> - Discussion of risk factors, potential complications, and management
> - Addressing questions

even part of one—causes significant problems. For example, having an extra chromosome 21 causes Down syndrome, in which there is intellectual disability and often major birth defects. Having an extra chromosome 13 or 18 is less common, but causes abnormalities which are often determined to be fatal for the fetus either during pregnancy, shortly after birth, or in the first year of life. Other chromosomal abnormalities have other outcomes, but all results can be discussed with a genetic counselor.

It has long been recognized that the risk of having a baby with a chromosomal abnormality such as Down syndrome increases with maternal age. Originally, genetic testing during pregnancy was only offered to women age 35 and older, when the risk of finding an abnormality was considered concerningly high. At the age of 35, the risk of the fetus having Down syndrome is still quite small at 1/294, or about 0.3%, with the risk of any type of chromosomal abnormality being 1/84, or about 1.2%. This risk doubles by age 40, with an increasingly larger jump every year after that (table 4.1). When looked at in this way it can be frightening; but looking at it differently a 40-year-old woman has a roughly 97.5% chance that the baby is chromosomally normal, and a 45-year-old woman conceiving

Table 4.1 Risk of Chromosomal Abnormalities by Maternal Age*

Maternal age at delivery	Risk of Down syndrome	Risk of any chromosomal abnormality
20	1/1250	1/122
25	1/1000	1/119
30	1/714	1/110
35	1/294	1/84
40	1/86	1/40
45	1/30	1/21

* For women conceiving with their own eggs.

Source: Committee on Clinical Consensus—Obstetric, Society for Maternal-Fetal Medicine. Pregnancy at age 35 years and older. *Obstet Gynecol* 2022; 140(2):348–366.

with her own eggs still has a 95% chance that the baby is chromosomally normal.

It is now recognized that 80% of babies with Down syndrome are born to women under age 35.[1] Standard care now includes offering genetic testing to all patients, regardless of age. The original way to test for a chromosomal abnormality was with amniocentesis. During this procedure, a needle is inserted into the mother's abdomen under ultrasound guidance, and fluid from around the baby is withdrawn and sent for testing. Soon after, CVS, or chorionic villus sampling, became available as an alternative, which involved taking a placental biopsy. Both tests involve a small risk of causing a miscarriage, well under 1%. However, CVS can be done about a month earlier than amniocentesis. Both tests are highly accurate and are, on occasion, still the best option.

Earlier in the pregnancy, there is a blood test available known as serum screening. Blood from the mother is not tested for fetal DNA but rather for levels of certain proteins or hormones that tend to increase or decrease with chromosomal abnormalities. It is sometimes referred to as sequential screening, or quad screening, and often is paired with an ultrasound to look for abnormal thickness at the back of the fetus's neck. This test is useful for patients at low risk for chromosomal abnormalities, but it only detects 90% of these abnormalities, and there are many false positives.

Over the past decade, blood tests have been developed that can detect chromosome abnormalities more accurately without any risk of losing the pregnancy from the procedure. These tests go by various names, including cell-free DNA testing and NIPT (non-invasive prenatal testing). Blood from the mother is tested for tiny fragments (cell-free fragments) of fetal DNA that get through the placenta and into the mother's circulation, looking for excess fetal DNA from a single chromosome. This test detects most whole chromosome abnormalities and is more accurate than serum screening but is not quite as accurate as the CVS or amniocentesis. Nonetheless, it is an appropriate option for those women who want a higher level of reassurance without the risk of a procedure, although some insurance plans may not cover it.

You might decide you need to know with certainty that the chromosomes are normal and opt for a CVS or amniocentesis, willing to take the very small risk of a problem from the procedure. Most likely you will get a normal result without any procedure-related complication. Or you might choose to have cell-free DNA testing, satisfied with the 98% accuracy and not taking any risk of losing the pregnancy from the procedure. Alternatively, you may choose not to have any genetic testing. There are some women who would not consider termination of the pregnancy if the result were abnormal, but still want to have the testing for the reassurance they will likely get from a normal result. You just need to decide which approach is best for you.

Whereas chromosomal abnormalities involve large segments or whole chromosomes, gene mutations occur when there may be as little as a single mistake in the DNA sequence, obstructing a gene's ability to work properly. All people have some gene mutations, but they are not a problem if there is a correct gene on the other chromosome of the pair, in which case the person is a carrier for that gene defect. However, if both parents are carriers of mutations in the same gene, there is a chance that the baby will receive both mutations and have a disease as a result. Examples of this are cystic fibrosis and sickle cell anemia. There are now blood tests that can be done to determine whether the mother is a carrier for over 200 single-gene abnormalities, and this test can be done before or during pregnancy. If you are the one in five women to have at least one of these 200 mutations, your partner should be tested to see if he has a mutation at the same gene. If not, the baby will be unaffected and at most an asymptomatic carrier like you.

Genetic testing is not mandatory, and many women choose not to do it. But if you want to test, it is important for you to know and understand your options and discuss them early on with your care provider. Genetic abnormalities that might be found will be discussed further in chapter 16.

SUMMARY

For women with high-risk issues, planning is important for optimizing pregnancy outcome. Women with underlying medical conditions should discuss their plans for conception with their caregiver to allow for assessment of condition control, blood testing that may be helpful, and any medication changes that should be made. Many things need to be done at the first prenatal visit, including confirming the pregnancy's viability, assignment of gestational age and a due date, identification of any additional high-risk factors that may be present, and reviewing the options for genetic testing. Plans for care for the pregnancy are outlined, and it is a great opportunity to ask questions. Just as important, the first prenatal visit is the time to establish a rapport with your caregiver, and make sure that you are comfortable with the evolving doctor-patient relationship.

CHAPTER 5

MISCARRIAGE

IT IS VERY EXCITING for a couple who are trying to conceive to first see a positive home pregnancy test. This urine test can be positive as early as two weeks after conception. Often women want to be seen by their obstetrician soon thereafter, but most offices want the patient to wait at least another two to three weeks before a first prenatal visit. This is because no testing needs to be done this early in the pregnancy, and it is too early to evaluate the pregnancy by ultrasound. By four weeks after conception (six weeks' gestation) the ultrasound can determine whether twins are present, whether the size confirms the presumed gestational age, and, usually, whether the fetal heart is beating. Unfortunately, sometimes the ultrasound may show that a pregnancy has already ended. Estimates vary between 10–15% as to what percentage of pregnancies end in miscarriage. After the maternal age of 35, the risk is even higher, reaching as high as 50% by age 45.[1]

DEFINITIONS

"Miscarriage" is a term often used for the loss of pregnancy before the end of the second trimester, but it is not a medical term. The medical term when it occurs before 20 weeks is a "spontaneous abortion." Sometimes a woman has a positive pregnancy test, but there is no sign of pregnancy in the uterus on ultrasound. This is often referred to as a chemical pregnancy. The woman will likely experience menstrual-like bleeding at or soon after her period is expected, and the pregnancy test turns to negative within a few days. If a fetus is seen on ultrasound, a spontaneous abortion can still happen, often through a series of stages. If bleeding starts but the pregnancy is still viable (still has a heart rate on ultrasound), it is referred to as a threatened abortion. Often this bleeding will stop within days, and a healthy pregnancy can still ensue. The longer this bleeding persists and the heavier it is, the worse the prognosis. If the cervix begins to open, spontaneous abortion is inevitable, and it will likely progress on its own. Once part of the pregnancy comes through the cervix, it is referred to as an incomplete abortion. The entire pregnancy may pass on its own, or an instrument can be inserted through the cervix into the uterus to remove any remaining tissue. When the entire pregnancy has come out of the uterus and the cervix is again closed, it is called a complete abortion. No further treatment is needed, and the woman will likely ovulate again in a few weeks.

When a pregnancy sac is present on ultrasound but no fetus is present, it is referred to as a blighted ovum. If a patient is asymptomatic but a fetus without a heartbeat is observed on ultrasound, it is referred to as a missed abortion. Unfortunately, these last two scenarios are not uncommon occurrences at first prenatal visits. Management of the blighted ovum and missed abortion are discussed later in this chapter. Although uncommon, a spontaneous abortion can still occur after a normal ultrasound at a first prenatal visit, but the further into pregnancy you go, the less likely this is to occur. Only 1–3% of pregnancies will spontaneously abort after the first trimester.

If this is your first pregnancy, the risk of a spontaneous abortion is roughly 1 in 5. If you have had four children and conceive again, the risk is also 1 in 5. If you have had one or two losses in a row, the risk in the subsequent pregnancy is still 1 in 5. So, 1 in 25 women will have a spontaneous abortion the first two times she conceives. Most likely this has occurred to at least one woman you know—it is not that rare. It is not until you have had at least three losses in a row that the odds begin to get worse than 1 in 5 for the next pregnancy.

CAUSES OF SPONTANEOUS ABORTION

The most common cause of spontaneous abortion is a genetic abnormality. Studies have demonstrated that chromosomal abnormalities are present in more than half of pregnancies that are lost in the first trimester, mostly with an extra whole chromosome, or trisomy. The older a woman is, the greater the chances are of a chromosomal abnormality being the cause. There are probably other types of genetic causes as well that are not currently identifiable. Types of chromosomal abnormalities seen with miscarriage can include an extra chromosome 13, 16, 18, 21, or 22, and monosomy X (only one sex chromosome instead of XX or XY). Even though babies born with trisomy 21 and monosomy X can live into adulthood, the majority spontaneously abort in the first trimester. While babies with trisomies 13 and 18 can be born alive, the majority also abort early in the pregnancy. With trisomy 16 and 22, the genetic information is so abnormal that rarely do these pregnancies make it out of the first trimester.

Chromosomal abnormalities occur at the time of conception—either a genetically abnormal sperm or a genetically abnormal egg was involved in fertilization. Chromosomal abnormalities occur to a large degree by random chance and nothing can be done to prevent them from occurring; it has nothing to do with anything the woman or man did before or after conception. As upsetting as this can be, it does not indicate a higher chance of future failed pregnancies or an inability to conceive.

Tissue obtained from a miscarriage can be sent for chromosomal analysis, and it often takes a few weeks for the results to be available. It should be recognized that in up to 50% of cases the results will be normal, and no cause for the miscarriage is identified. It may be that a different type of genetic abnormality other than a missing or extra whole chromosome is present and responsible for the loss, but these other types of genetic abnormalities remain largely unknown.

Other issues that can contribute to risk of spontaneous abortion are uterine abnormalities, some chronic medical conditions, a hormonal deficiency, and some viral illnesses. Uterine structural anomalies can be identified in a number of ways, including ultrasound and magnetic resonance imaging (MRI). A uterine septum (discussed in chapter 13) increases the chances of miscarriage, and if found, can be removed with an instrument inserted through the cervix. Poorly controlled diabetes and thyroid disease can also increase the risk of miscarriage. Progesterone deficiency has also been implicated in recurrent pregnancy loss. However, since these causes are so uncommon, it is not usually recommended that they should be investigated until a woman has experienced three or more spontaneous losses, when the likelihood of finding a problem begins to increase. In the second trimester, if a loss is preceded by cervical dilation without contractions and the fetus still has a heartbeat, this may suggest a condition known as cervical insufficiency. This will be discussed further in chapter 26.

MANAGEMENT OF SPONTANEOUS ABORTION

When a woman begins to bleed in the early stages of pregnancy, it can be a cause for concern. The first step at this point would be to perform an ultrasound. Understandably, a bleeding pregnant woman will want this done as soon as possible. But as long as the bleeding is not excessive, the situation is not urgent; waiting for your caregiver's office to open the next day may save you waiting for hours in an emergency room as more acutely ill patients are cared for first. Once a spontaneous abortion has been diagnosed, a discussion can be had as to how it should be managed. Nothing needs to be done if the abortion is complete. For all other stages, waiting to see if the pregnancy passes completely on its own is always an option unless you are hemorrhaging, which is exceedingly rare. If the patient is bleeding and cramping with an inevitable or incomplete abortion, often the process of miscarriage will be complete within 24 hours without any medical intervention, though you should notify your doctor if anything seems amiss.

With a blighted ovum or missed abortion, the time course is more uncertain, and some patients can go days or even weeks without developing symptoms and passing the pregnancy. For patients who do not want to wait for the spontaneous abortion to complete on its own, there are options. One is a D&C, or dilation and curettage, a minor procedure under local anesthesia which involves use of instruments to remove any parts of the pregnancy that remain in the uterus. Another option may be what is sometimes referred to as a medical abortion, where pills are taken to hasten the uterus's expulsion of the pregnancy. For inevitable and incomplete abortions that do not progress to complete abortion, the options of curettage and medication are also available.

NEXT STEPS

After miscarriage, what should you do? The first thing is to recover physically and emotionally. For most women, physical recovery is not difficult, and many are back to routine activities within a week. There can be cramping, especially after a medical abortion, but it should resolve within a few days. But if bleeding or cramping persist, notify your care provider. Some physicians recommend a follow-up visit a few weeks after, but this is mainly to address any questions you may still have. Recovering emotionally may take longer. Some women go through a grieving process, and support from family and friends can be very helpful in this regard. Not only can there be profound disappointment after the excitement of expecting a child, but also fear that future attempts at pregnancy will end similarly. Hopefully, the statistics provided in this chapter will give you reason for optimism, that the odds for a future successful pregnancy are very much in your favor.

A frequent question asked after miscarriage is "How long do I need to wait before trying again?" Traditionally, physicians have counseled patients to wait three to six months to allow them to recover both physically and emotionally. However, this recommendation is without supporting data. You may say that the thing that will help most in your emotional recovery would be to be pregnant again. The best time for you to conceive is when you feel you are ready, but any medical conditions that have not yet been optimized should be addressed first.

SUMMARY

First-trimester miscarriage is a common event that can occur to any woman unrelated to underlying conditions. Most are caused by chromosomal abnormalities, which occur frequently. After one or even two miscarriages, the prognosis is still quite good that the next pregnancy will not have the same result. If you experience bleeding or any symptoms that seem out of the realm of normal to you, it is best to contact your health care practitioner to discuss, even just to put your mind at ease.

PART III

MATERNAL CONDITIONS

CHAPTER 6

HYPERTENSION

IF YOU HAVE HIGH BLOOD PRESSURE in pregnancy, you are not alone. Hypertension is the most common preexisting chronic condition affecting women entering pregnancy. And like many other conditions, its frequency has been rising. Birth certificate data from the year 2000 listed 0.76% of mothers having chronic hypertension, while similar data from 2021 has the frequency of preexisting hypertension at 2.8%. The statistics are worse for Black Americans, with the 2021 frequency being 4.9%.[1] Why the numbers are rising is not completely clear, but it is likely related to increasing rates of obesity and age at which women are having babies. The causes of hypertension are not well understood, but the frequency of it occurring within families points to genetics as a major factor. Most women with hypertension are asymptomatic, so the diagnosis is sometimes made at a first prenatal visit if the patient has not had routine primary care.

Blood pressure readings consist of two numbers separated by a forward slash (/). The first number is the systolic reading, when the pressure of the blood flow is the highest, and the second is the diastolic, when the pressure of the blood flow is the lowest. Traditionally readings less than 140/90 were considered normal, but now normal is defined as 120/80 or lower. Systolic blood pressure of

120–129 is now considered elevated, and 130s/80s is now considered stage 1 hypertension.

Having high blood pressure for decades can lead to damage to the heart, kidneys, eyes, and blood vessels, as well as increasing the risk of stroke. Fortunately, these complications are very uncommon in women in their reproductive years, unless the blood pressure has been poorly controlled for many years. Diet, exercise, and medication are the cornerstones for controlling hypertension prior to pregnancy, and during pregnancy as well.

CLASSIFICATION OF HYPERTENSIVE DISORDERS IN PREGNANCY

Hypertension in pregnancy is now classified into four categories: chronic hypertension, gestational hypertension, preeclampsia-eclampsia, and preeclampsia superimposed on chronic hypertension. While not every woman will fit neatly into one of these categories, the classification system works for most pregnant women. *Chronic hypertension* is used for patients with persistent blood pressure greater than 140/90 diagnosed before pregnancy or first noted in pregnancy before 20 weeks. It also is used retrospectively for those women whose hypertension is first observed during pregnancy and persists beyond 12 weeks after delivery. *Gestational hypertension* is new-onset elevations of blood pressure after 20 weeks of gestation in women who do not meet the criteria for preeclampsia. If gestational hypertension persists long after delivery, the diagnosis is then changed to chronic hypertension. *Preeclampsia* is new-onset hypertension after 20 weeks' gestation with proteinuria (significant elevation of protein in the urine) or other signs discussed in chapter 22, and eclampsia is when a patient with preeclampsia develops seizures. Preeclampsia superimposed on chronic hypertension is just as it sounds—when a woman with underlying chronic hypertension develops additional signs of preeclampsia. The rest of this chapter will focus on chronic hypertension and gestational hypertension, with preeclampsia addressed in chapter 22.

RISKS ASSOCIATED WITH HYPERTENSION DURING PREGNANCY

The risks associated with hypertension during pregnancy extend to both the mother and the fetus. Although it is still very uncommon, the mother with hypertension is at least five times more likely to have a stroke, renal failure, and death compared to women with normal blood pressure.[2] The increased frequency and severity of hypertension seen in African American women is a leading cause for the disparity in maternal mortality between races. The chances of a major complication are difficult to predict by blood pressure alone, yet those with pressures consistently above 160/105 are at the highest risk. These risks are reduced significantly if the blood pressure is well controlled with medication.

The risks to the fetus correlate with the degree of hypertension in the mother. These risks include poor fetal growth, placental abruption (detachment of the placenta from the uterus, chapter 23), need for preterm delivery, and perinatal death. As with maternal risk, the fetal risk is reduced significantly if the blood pressure is well controlled. To further reduce fetal risk, "fetal surveillance" is routinely recommended in the third trimester. This surveillance can be in the form of a non-stress test (NST) or biophysical profile (BPP) starting around 32 weeks of gestation. For the NST, a monitor is placed on the mother's abdomen over the fetal heart, and it records the fetal heart rate for 20–30 minutes. The pattern of this fetal heart rate is then interpreted as either reassuring or non-reassuring. If non-reassuring, further testing is performed to determine whether the fetal condition is actually deteriorating and the fetus would be better off being delivered. The BPP is performed with ultrasound and examines fetal behavior and activities which are indicative of being healthy. These behaviors include body movements, flexion and extension of the arms and legs, the amount of amniotic fluid around the fetus (as a reflection of normal kidney function), and fetal breathing movements. Yes, the fetus actually inhales and exhales fluid inside the uterus before birth, and the movement of the diaphragm is easily seen with ultrasound. Seeing the presence of these behaviors is a sign of a well-oxygenated fetus and should be reassuring. However, missing two or more behaviors warrants further investigation, and early delivery may be needed to avoid stillbirth. These tests of fetal well-being are also used for other maternal and fetal conditions which may put the fetus in jeopardy, and will be discussed again in parts III and IV. For most situations with concern for fetal well-being, either the NST or the BPP is performed at least weekly until the time of delivery.

MANAGEMENT OF HYPERTENSION DURING PREGNANCY

With hypertension, the goal of therapy is primarily for you to avoid having blood pressure readings of 160/105 or higher. Ideally, you want to have readings with the systolic number 130-140/80-90. Although this range is now considered to be hypertensive, being in this range for the nine months of pregnancy will not have a major impact on your long-term health. If medication takes the blood pressure below 120/70, it may increase the chances of the fetus developing growth restriction (chapter 18).

Some women with hypertension will spontaneously experience a drop in their blood pressure toward the end of the first trimester, and they made need a reduction in the pre-pregnancy medication dose to keep pressure from getting too low. For these women, the blood pressure will then rise in the second half of pregnancy, and the dose may then need to be increased. For other women, blood pressure may be unchanged or may even increase in early pregnancy, and dose adjustments should be made accordingly. It is not uncommon for women with hypertension to need their dose adjusted more than once during the pregnancy.

Blood pressure medications are best discussed in "classes." One class of medications often used outside of pregnancy are called ACE inhibitors, and another is angiotensin receptor blockers (ARBs). These are very effective medications, but they are not used during pregnancy because of concern that they will interfere with the kidney development in the fetus. Diuretics are another class of medications that are useful outside of pregnancy, but usually not used during pregnancy. If a woman on these medications becomes pregnant, she is usually switched to another agent. Some primary care doctors will switch a patient to methyl dopa, but most obstetricians prefer to use more effective agents. The most recommended classes of antihypertensive agents for pregnancy are beta blockers and calcium channel blockers. There is a lot of experience with these medications in pregnancy over the years, which supports their effectiveness and safety with few side effects. Examples of frequently used medications are labetalol (beta blocker) and nifedipine (calcium channel blocker). If your blood pressure is more severe, you may need to take both, and even have a third agent added, but this is very uncommon. It is recommended that patients with chronic hypertension also take a single low- dose aspirin tablet (81 mg) once a day beginning at the end of the first trimester to decrease the chances of developing superimposed preeclampsia.

Even when the blood pressure is controlled, you need to be monitored for appropriate fetal growth with ultrasound. In addition, tests of fetal well-being are usually initiated at 32–34 weeks.

CASE STUDY #1

Latrice was a 34-year-old woman who presented for her first prenatal visit at nine weeks' gestation with a strong family history of hypertension. Latrice was diagnosed with hypertension herself at age 24 and initially started on a diuretic and a low-sodium diet. At age 31 it was decided that her blood pressure was not being adequately controlled on the diuretic and she was switched to lisinopril (an ACE inhibitor) with good effect. She had no evidence of other vascular disease and her kidney function was normal. At this visit her blood pressure was 146/96; she was told to stop the lisinopril and start taking nifedipine 30 mg daily as well as a low-dose aspirin tablet. She began recording her blood pressure readings twice a day at home. After two weeks, blood pressure readings were still mostly above 140/90, and the nifedipine dose was increased to 60 mg daily. This dose helped to maintain most readings under 140/90, and she continued it through the end of the second trimester.

At 27 weeks her blood pressure elevated further, with many readings above 150/100. The nifedipine dose was increased to 90 mg daily, and then 120 mg daily at 31 weeks. Ultrasound of the fetus revealed fetal growth at the 10th percentile, and weekly fetal surveillance with non-stress testing (NSTs) was initiated. At her office visit at 33 weeks, her blood pressure was noted to be 155/102, and now with significant proteinuria. She was admitted to the hospital for assessment of possible superimposed preeclampsia, and labetalol 200 mg twice a day was added to the nifedipine for blood pressure control. At 34 weeks, it was decided that the risks to the mother of the hypertension with superimposed preeclampsia was a greater risk than prematurity was to the fetus, and delivery was recommended. Induction of labor was successful, and she delivered a 4-pound baby girl vaginally without complications. However, after delivery blood pressure control was difficult to maintain, and a diuretic was added to the maximum doses of nifedipine and labetalol to achieve blood pressures consistently less than 150/100. She was discharged on day six after delivery. The baby had mild issues with prematurity and was discharged in *good condition at three weeks of life. Latrice was able to stop one of her blood pressure medications after one month, and by three months was back on her lisinopril at her pre-pregnancy dose.*

CASE STUDY #2

Paula was a 29-year-old woman in her first pregnancy with no history of medical problems prior to pregnancy. At her first prenatal visit, her blood pressure was normal, and no other abnormalities were noted. She came for monthly visits after this, and was noted to be doing well until her visit at 33 weeks, when she had her first elevated blood pressure of 148/94. Laboratory tests showed a normal platelet count and normal liver function tests, and her urine showed only trace protein. An ultrasound demonstrated a fetus growing at the 60th percentile, and an NST showed reassuring fetal status. A plan was made for Paula to record her blood pressure at home twice a day and to report any readings above 150/100, changes in her vision, or development of a headache (potential signs of preeclampsia).

Paula returned to the office in one week, with all of her blood pressure readings 130–150/80–100, and denied any concerning symptoms. The fetus was still normally active, and her NST was again reassuring. Her office BP reading was 142/96, and her urine was negative for protein. Her laboratory tests remained normal. A diagnosis of gestational hypertension was made, with no change in the plan for daily home blood pressure monitoring and symptom surveillance, and weekly office visits with laboratory tests and NSTs.

At 37 weeks, Paula's home blood pressure readings began to increase, with multiple readings now in the 150s/90s. In the office her blood pressure was similarly elevated, and when repeated was 160/102 on one occasion. Her laboratory results were still in the normal range without significant proteinuria. However, because the risk of her worsening gestational hypertension was now thought to be greater than the risk to the fetus of prematurity, a decision was made to move to delivery. She was admitted to the hospital for labor induction, and 20 hours later delivered a healthy male infant weighing 8 pounds. Over the next few days, Paula's blood pressure returned to normal, and was back to her baseline level at her office visit six weeks later taking no medication.

SUMMARY

Hypertension is a common high-risk issue during pregnancy and often needs close attention to maintain adequate blood pressure control. Some women do very well and have no complications, while others may need increasing doses of medication and early delivery. Either way, the prognosis is still very good that there will be a good outcome for the baby without any effect on the mother's long-term health. Attention to blood pressure control needs to continue after delivery to ensure that it returns to normal.

CHAPTER 7

DIABETES

OVER THE PAST 40 YEARS, the prevalence of diabetes in the United States has increased significantly in all age groups, including in women of child-bearing age. Much of this increase has been attributed to the rise in overweight and obesity, but other factors exist. Management of diabetes during pregnancy can be a challenge, but a challenge that most women can meet.

If you have diabetes, the most important thing to focus on is blood sugar control. Glucose is the main type of sugar in the bloodstream; therefore, its control is important from before conception until after delivery. The absence of good blood sugar (glycemic) control is associated with an increased risk of pregnancy complications including birth defects, miscarriage, maternal ketoacidosis (dangerously high levels of glucose), fetal death, preeclampsia, abnormally large fetal growth (macrosomia), and fetal injury during delivery. For most people, optimal glycemic control will be achieved through a combination of diet, exercise, and insulin therapy.

HISTORY OF DIABETES DURING PREGNANCY

Insulin was first discovered about 100 years ago, but it was some years after that before it was widely available for patients with diabetes. Until then, women with diabetes were rarely able to have a family. Even with early insulin treatment, those with diabetes had a high rate of miscarriage due to difficulties controlling blood sugar throughout the day, leading to frequent episodes of elevated blood sugar (hyperglycemia). Even if miscarriage did not occur, this population had a very high rate of stillbirth. The first method of self-testing for people with diabetes seems relatively crude by today's standards, as patients would use color-coded test strips to assess glucose levels in their urine. Since urine stays in the bladder for hours before urination, this type of testing assessed one's average blood sugar from hours before, rendering measurements less reflective of *current* levels. It wasn't until the 1970s that finger-stick testing was introduced to assess current blood sugar levels to determine the appropriate insulin dosage. Because of the high rate of adverse pregnancy outcomes, women with diabetes were frequently admitted to the hospital for many weeks or even months prior to delivery to improve glycemic control and perform daily testing of fetal well-being. When concerns for fetal deterioration arose, early delivery was performed, often resulting in a baby with complications of prematurity.

With significant advances in the 1980s and early 1990s, expectant mothers could monitor their blood sugars at home with finger-sticks and meters, and no longer needed routine hospitalization. Rates of complications dropped, and most women were able to carry their pregnancies to term and have healthy babies with few issues in the newborn period. There were still some women, however, who entered pregnancy already with complications of long-term diabetes, such as kidney disease, hypertension, and vascular disease. For these women, pregnancy was still challenging, and complications were more frequent.

Today, pregnancy for women with diabetes is routinely better, as few women enter pregnancy with diabetic complications. And most women can have as many children as they desire without it affecting their long-term prognosis for diabetes complications. Yet, good glycemic control is still very important. Many women now have access to insulin pumps and continuous glucose monitors, which makes glycemic control much easier and helps avoid unrecognized periods of hyperglycemia.

TYPES OF DIABETES: TYPE I, TYPE II, AND GESTATIONAL DIABETES

Patients with diabetes are routinely divided into those with type I diabetes and those with type II. Type I is often referred to as juvenile-onset, although it can have an onset in adulthood. It is caused by antibodies forming in the body that attack insulin-producing cells in the pancreas. Unable to make sufficient insulin, the body cannot remove carbohydrates from the bloodstream after eating, and blood sugar levels rise. Over many years, this hyperglycemia can lead to diabetic complications, including kidney disease, eye disease, and vascular complications.

Type II diabetes is often referred to as adult-onset, but it is now seen more frequently in teenagers. It is often related to obesity and can improve with weight loss and proper diet. In type II diabetes, the problem is insulin resistance—the pancreas makes insulin, but because of factors in the body causing resistance, the insulin is insufficient to achieve glycemic control. Over many years, this hyperglycemia of type II diabetes can also lead to the same types of diabetic complications: kidney disease, eye disease, and vascular complications.

Gestational diabetes is diagnosed when hyperglycemia is first identified during pregnancy in a patient who was not diabetic prior to conception. It is currently recommended that all patients be screened for gestational diabetes after 24 weeks of gestation, with a blood glucose level taken after drinking a liquid that contains a specific amount of carbohydrates. In normal pregnancy, at around 20 weeks of gestation the placenta begins to produce a hormone called HPL in increasing quantities, and HPL increases insulin resistance. Most women can still maintain glycemic control despite the HPL increase, but those with gestational diabetes cannot, and by 24 weeks this is evident. A carbohydrate-limited diet is often sufficient to control gestational diabetes, but some women need either oral medication or insulin to achieve control. After pregnancy, gestational diabetes resolves for most women, but they are at increased risk of being diagnosed with type II diabetes within the next five years.

RISKS ASSOCIATED WITH DIABETES DURING PREGNANCY

The first risk to discuss related to diabetes is birth defects. For the general population, the risk of having a fetus with a major birth defect is 2.5%, or 1 in every 40 babies. This is higher than most people realize. Even with good glycemic control, that risk doubles for patients with diabetes; with poor control the risk increases to 10–20%.[1] Most birth defects form beginning around 3–5 weeks after conception, before many women realize they are pregnant. Since it often takes weeks to get blood sugar under control it is best to focus on and achieve control of your blood sugar before conception (box 7.1).

The most common birth defects seen in infants of diabetic mothers are heart defects. Many of these cardiac malformations are severe enough to require heart surgery after the baby is born. Amazingly, with today's surgical capabilities, most babies having corrective heart surgery go on to lead normal lives. In fact, many high-risk obstetric practices are now seeing pregnant women who had open heart surgery as infants. Advances in prenatal ultrasound now make it possible to identify more than 80% of all cardiac defects by 18–20 weeks of gestation. Because of the higher rate of cardiac defects in this population, physicians often refer patients with diabetes to a pediatric cardiologist to perform a fetal heart echo, or fetal echocardiogram, to look more closely for heart malformations.

Other fetal anomalies more often found in the infants of patients with diabetes include abnormalities of the spine and kidneys, among other organs. Given the overall increased risk of anomalies, more extensive examinations are performed using targeted ultrasound, or level II ultrasound. A targeted ultrasound examines more views of the brain, heart, and limbs. As such, if you have a targeted ultrasound that does not identify any abnormalities, it should be very reassuring.

BOX 7.1 RISKS ASSOCIATED WITH DIABETES IN PREGNANCY

- Birth defects
    - Congenital heart defects
    - Neural tube defects
    - Kidney abnormalities
- Fetal death
- Fetal macrosomia
- Preeclampsia
- Cesarean delivery
- Neonatal hypoglycemia

Women with diabetes are also at increased risk for a fetus that dies before delivery, or stillbirth. This was far more common in the days before routine daily glucose monitoring improved glucose control, but it is still of concern, especially in a patient with poor control or episodes of ketoacidosis. To reduce this risk, initiating a form of fetal surveillance in the third trimester is routinely recommended. This can be with an NST or BPP, as described in chapter 6.

Another risk for expectant mothers with diabetes is macrosomia, where the estimated fetal size is greater than the 90th percentile. Which means, typically, patients with diabetes have bigger babies. This is especially true when glycemic control is suboptimal. The excess glucose in the mother's blood easily crosses the placenta into the circulation of the fetus, raising its blood sugar level. Since there is nothing wrong with the fetal pancreas, it makes more insulin to handle this increased load. In addition to regulating blood sugar, insulin acts as an important growth factor in the fetus. So increased maternal glucose levels lead to increased levels of insulin in the fetus, and then increased growth. But this is not necessarily healthy growth and may contribute to later development of obesity in the child. Infant size does not always correlate with maternal glucose control, as many women with well-controlled blood sugar still have large babies. The larger infant may have a harder time fitting through the pelvis, so the rate of cesarean birth is increased. There is also a higher rate of a complication known as shoulder dystocia for vaginal birth of infants of diabetic mothers, especially if the newborn weighs more than 10 pounds. Shoulder dystocia occurs when the head of the baby delivers but the shoulders are stuck in the pelvis. Special maneuvers are then needed to deliver the child without causing injury to the nerves in the neck. Occasionally, the news media reports on a baby born larger than 13 pounds as a human interest story. This should be viewed not as a media event but as an unhealthy situation and one with significant risk to the infant.

As mentioned previously, women with diabetes are at increased risk for developing preeclampsia. When this occurs, it may require maternal hospitalization and early delivery. The infant of a diabetic mother tends to have delayed lung maturation compared with other infants, so premature delivery in a diabetic patient may lead to more neonatal complications for a given gestational age. In a situation where premature delivery is anticipated, steroids will often be administered to the mother to accelerate the maturity of the infant's lungs, but the steroids frequently cause significant hyperglycemia in the mother, which can last for days despite efforts to control it with additional insulin. Jaundice, a situation where the baby's skin has a yellow color, is also more common for infants with diabetic mothers, and may prolong the baby's stay in the hospital. And paradoxically, after delivery the infant of a diabetic mother is at increased risk of developing hypoglycemia, or low blood sugar, within a few hours of delivery. When the umbilical cord is cut, the transfer of glucose from the mother ends, but the insulin made by the fetus remains in the system driving the newborn's blood sugar down. To avoid the consequences of hypoglycemia, this infant may require early feeding or even intravenous glucose to maintain its blood sugar level until excess levels of insulin decrease to the normal range. This may take a few days and prolong the infant's stay in the hospital, but it does not have long-term consequences if the infant's blood sugar level is brought up to the normal range.

OBSTETRICAL MANAGEMENT OF DIABETES DURING PREGNANCY

Maintaining normal glycemia before and during pregnancy is the most important thing you can do to reduce the risks associated with diabetes in pregnancy. The best measure of overall diabetes control is your blood level of hemoglobin A1c. Hemoglobin is the oxygen-carrying molecule in red blood cells, and glucose attaches to hemoglobin. A1c levels assess the percentage of RBCs (red blood cells) that have glucose attached, and this reflects average blood sugar levels over the last 1–3 months. The higher average blood sugar levels are, the higher the A1c. People without diabetes have A1c levels of 5.6% or less, and for patients with diabetes in good control the A1c level is usually between 6% and 7%. Ideally, as a diabetic patient you should have an A1c level less than 7% prior to conception and maintain this level throughout the pregnancy. This is tighter control than you are probably used to, and may require you to work with a dietician and a diabetic specialist to achieve this level of control. If it is achieved, however, you will likely be in the best control since your diagnosis, and if you can maintain this after pregnancy, it will be beneficial for your long-term health.

The first trimester can be quite difficult for some patients with diabetes. The nausea and vomiting that some experience can interfere with eating, and the pregnancy also extracts glucose from the system. Together, these phenomena can lead to episodes of hypoglycemia, and insulin doses may need to be reduced. Hypoglycemia episodes can be dangerous for the mother, but fortunately, rarely is harmful to the fetus. Like patients with chronic hypertension and some other conditions, it is routinely recommended that women with diabetes also take a single low-dose aspirin tablet daily beginning at 12–16 weeks, which is thought to reduce the risk of developing preeclampsia.

During the second trimester things get somewhat easier as the early symptoms of nausea and tiredness usually dissipate. Other than continued attention to glycemic control, no testing or interventions are routine until the ultrasound examination at 18–20 weeks. This ultrasound, which checks for anomalies, is not usually done sooner because the fetal structures need to grow big enough to distinguish normal from abnormal. For some patients even this is too early, and an ultrasound needs to be repeated a few weeks later to obtain all of the desired views when the fetus is larger. As stated previously, you will likely see your blood sugars rising after 20 weeks due to placental hormone production, and your insulin needs will begin to rise. This rise in insulin requirements routinely continues until the end of pregnancy, and is not a sign of a problem.

As you enter the third trimester, medical visits usually increase in frequency. Periodic ultrasounds are performed to assess fetal growth, and weekly fetal surveillance (NSTs or BPPs) begins at 32 weeks of gestation. At some time between 32 and 36 weeks, plans for delivery and your preferences will be addressed. At this time, you may choose to discuss epidural anesthesia for labor, as well as possible methods of delivery. Vaginal delivery is safe and preferable unless the fetus is thought to be unusually large. Delivery by your due date is preferable, as the concerns for fetal well-being after that can outweigh the benefits of spontaneous labor.

During labor, efforts are made to control maternal blood sugar through frequent glucose testing, but otherwise labor management is no different than for patients without diabetes. After delivery, tight glucose control is not as necessary, and insulin needs drop quickly. It is not uncommon for the daily dose of insulin a patient needs right after delivery to be at or below what they took prior to pregnancy. Breastfeeding is recommended, and this also helps to reduce insulin requirements.

If you are diagnosed with gestational diabetes at or after 24 weeks, you are initially placed on a carbohydrate-limited diet. The caloric needs are met with an increase in protein intake. Blood sugar testing is initiated at either one or two hours after eating, and before eating in the morning. If diet changes are insufficient to control blood sugar either after an overnight fast or after meals, medication will be introduced. Some physicians begin with oral medication while others move directly to insulin injections. Oral medication is cheaper and easier to take, but insulin injections are often superior in controlling blood sugar levels. If either medication is used, fetal monitoring is usually recommended, and the remainder of the pregnancy is managed as it is for patients with type I or type II diabetes as described above. However, after delivery women with gestational diabetes usually no longer need medication. Nonetheless, a glucose tolerance test should be performed six or more weeks after delivery to confirm that there is no persisting diabetes. It is important to note that even if this test for diabetes is negative, you still will be at increased risk for developing diabetes in the next few years. Losing weight and exercising may help avoid a diagnosis of overt diabetes in the future.

CASE STUDY #1

Jeanette was 26 years old and early in her first pregnancy. She was diagnosed with type I diabetes at age 8 and has been on insulin since. She had an episode of ketoacidosis at the time of diagnosis, but none since. Two years previously, she switched from insulin self-injections to an insulin pump and now wears a continuous glucose monitor (CGM), which she checks regularly. She does not stick to her recommended diabetic diet all the time but programs her pump for extra insulin on occasions when she has more carbohydrates or dessert. She had her eyes examined six months ago and there was no evidence of diabetic changes to her retinas. Six months ago, her A1c level was 7.4%, but she has been working with a diabetes specialist in preparation for pregnancy and her most recent level was 6.4%.

Jeanette was excited about being pregnant, but very anxious given the risks involved. She continued to work with the diabetes specialist and by 18 weeks her A1c was 5.9%. The ultrasound at 20 weeks found no fetal anomalies, and the fetal cardiac echo was normal—which relieved her anxiety quite a bit. She continued to maintain her A1c around 6.0%, but the ultrasound at 30 weeks' gestation suggested that the fetus was at the 90th percentile for size.

Weekly fetal surveillance with NSTs began at 32 weeks and all were reassuring. At 37 weeks, ultrasound again suggested that the baby was bigger than average and predicted a birth weight of around 9 pounds at term. She was scheduled for a labor induction five days before her due date. Labor lasted almost 24 hours, not unusual for a first pregnancy. During the labor her blood sugar was checked regularly and maintained in the normal range. After two hours of pushing, she delivered a healthy female infant vaginally weighing 8 pounds, 9 ounces. The baby developed mild hypoglycemia two hours after birth, which responded to a single feeding with formula. She began breastfeeding, and the mother and baby were discharged two days after delivery.

CASE STUDY #2

Linda was 32 years old when she had her first prenatal appointment in her second pregnancy. In her first pregnancy three years before, she was diagnosed with gestational diabetes, and insulin was prescribed after diet failed to control her hyperglycemia. She had a cesarean at 39 weeks after an ultrasound suggested that the birth weight would be over 10 pounds. The infant had significant hypoglycemia, which could not be alleviated by breastfeeding and formula, so IV glucose was given for the first three days of life. Linda's milk came in on the third day, and breastfeeding was then sufficient to maintain the baby's blood sugar in the normal range without additional IV glucose. She recovered normally from her cesarean, but testing six weeks after delivery showed continued elevation of her fasting and after meal blood sugars, giving Linda the diagnosis of type II diabetes. She was started on oral medication for this diabetes, and glucose values improved.

At her first prenatal visit in the second pregnancy, Linda's A1c level was 6.8%. She was told to stop the current diabetes medication and instructed on the use of an insulin pump and continuous glucose monitor. She was counseled about the risks of diabetes in pregnancy and the importance of glycemic control, and she met with a dietitian to discuss meal planning and snacks. By her office visit at 14 weeks, her A1c level was down to 6.1%. She continued to monitor her glucose levels and follow her diabetic diet for the remainder of the pregnancy. The targeted ultrasound at 20 weeks showed no anomalies, and the fetal echo performed by the pediatric cardiologist showed normal heart anatomy and function. Despite continued good glycemic control, periodic ultrasounds showed the baby growing above the 90th percentile for weight, and a repeat cesarean was performed at 39 weeks. The baby girl weighed 9½ pounds at birth and did not have issues with hypoglycemia, and was discharged with Linda three days after delivery. Linda received follow-up care for her diabetes with her primary care physician.

SUMMARY

Despite the potential risks, the prognosis for a healthy pregnancy for almost all women with diabetes is excellent. If you have diabetes, you should not be discouraged from becoming pregnant, and family size need not be limited. A discussion with your health care team regarding your desire to get pregnant will allow you to get a head start on management. Attention to good glucose control before and during pregnancy remains the best way to improve the chances of a successful outcome for you and your baby. Compared with nondiabetic women, a lot more is asked of you in terms of frequent blood sugar testing, appropriate diet, and more office visits and testing. Yet this extra effort is needed to maintain your health throughout pregnancy and optimize the chances of having a healthy baby.

CHAPTER 8

THYROID DISEASE

YOU MAY NOT KNOW much about your thyroid gland, but it has a very important role for proper body functioning. It sits in the front of your neck just above your collarbone. Its only purpose is to secrete hormones, the most important of which is thyroxine (also referred to as thyroid hormone). Thyroxine regulates metabolism in the body, so that an elevated level of thyroxine (hyperthyroidism) can cause a rapid heart rate, tremors, anxiety, weight loss, and heat intolerance. Low levels of thyroxine (hypothyroidism) can result in the opposite effect—fatigue, weight gain, cold intolerance, and a slowed heart rate. Hyperthyroidism (also known as Grave's disease) is five times more common in women than in men, with symptoms most commonly beginning between ages 20 and 40. The main risk factor is a family history of Grave's disease. Hypothyroidism is also more common in women, affecting around 5% of women in their reproductive years. Problems with the immune system are most often the cause of both hyper- and hypothyroidism, where different autoantibodies (proteins the body makes that attack its own organs) either stimulate or suppress thyroxine production. Both hyper- and hypothyroidism can cause infertility, and both can be a problem during pregnancy.

The pituitary gland in the brain exerts control over the thyroid gland. It secretes a hormone called thyroid stimulating hormone (TSH), which signals the thyroid to produce thyroxine. If thyroxine is overproduced, as in hyperthyroidism, TSH levels decrease in response. If the thyroid is underproducing thyroxine, the pituitary gland releases more TSH in an effort to correct the problem. Thus, measuring the level of TSH in the blood is a good screening test for both hyper- and hypothyroidism.

HYPERTHYROIDISM

In some ways, pregnancy has features which can mimic hyperthyroidism. By the second trimester, maternal heart rate is elevated 10–20 beats per minute, and many women begin to feel warmer than usual. The only way to make the diagnosis of hyperthyroidism is with a blood test showing an elevated level of thyroid hormone production. When identified, hyperthyroidism is first treated with medication. Methimazole (Tapazole) is one such drug, easing symptoms by reducing the amount of thyroxine the thyroid produces. Beta blockers such as labetalol do not decrease the amount of thyroxine produced, but they help to control the symptoms. If you are on methimazole prior to pregnancy, it will likely be switched to propylthiouracil (PTU) for the first trimester, and switched back to methimazole after that because of concerns that methimazole might cause birth defects if taken in early pregnancy. Longer-term usage of PTU can cause liver problems for the mother. Some patients eventually have their thyroid gland ablated with radioactive iodine, which selectively destroys the thyroxine-producing cells in the thyroid without effects on any other organs. But radioactive iodine cannot be given during pregnancy. Occasionally, surgical removal of the thyroid gland is performed. After either of these procedures, patients will need to take thyroxine pills to achieve a normal level. These people will no longer have any hyperthyroid symptoms but will still have the circulating antibodies, which have no effect.

When considering the effects of hyperthyroidism during pregnancy, it is important to understand the workings of the fetal thyroid. In the first trimester, the fetal thyroid produces little if any thyroid hormone, and is dependent upon the transfer of hormone from the mother to achieve normal levels. By the second trimester, the fetal thyroid begins to produce sufficient hormone for its needs. Methimazole, PTU, and beta blockers all cross the placenta, so if the mother is hyperthyroid and transfers excess thyroxine to the fetus, the medication will also transfer and prevent a problem with the fetus. For a woman who has had her thyroid ablated or surgically removed, she may now have a normal level of thyroid hormone with medication treatment, but the antibodies which originally caused her disease can still cross the placenta and overstimulate the fetal thyroid. This rarely happens, but could be the issue if the fetus is noted to have a faster than normal heart rate, or an enlarged neck seen on ultrasound.

HYPOTHYROIDISM

Hypothyroidism is diagnosed when blood testing shows an elevation in TSH and a low level of thyroxine, a sign of an underactive thyroid. Testing for hypothyroidism is not part of routine prenatal laboratory tests, but some doctors test for it during pregnancy, even if a patient is asymptomatic. Testing is indicated for women with type I diabetes, a family history of thyroid disease, or symptoms. For those diagnosed with hypothyroidism prior to pregnancy, taking thyroid hormone replacement is essential. The fetus depends on maternal thyroxine in the early part of pregnancy for normal brain development and growth. If oral thyroxine supplementation is needed to make up for inadequate maternal production, maternal blood levels of TSH should be checked periodically, as the dosage may need to be increased as the pregnancy progresses. The vast majority of women with treated hypothyroidism do not have pregnancy complications, and the baby is expected to be unaffected.

Some controversy exists regarding the entity called *subclinical hypothyroidism*. This is when TSH levels are elevated, but thyroxine levels are in the normal range. All patients in this situation are asymptomatic. Some endocrinologists feel that these women should be treated during pregnancy to bring their TSH levels back to normal in order to protect the brain of the fetus. This is based on some studies showing an association between subclinical hypothyroidism and pregnancy loss, gestational diabetes, preeclampsia, and preterm delivery. However, these findings are not found consistently in all studies. Further, two large prospective trials[1] of treatment for subclinical hypothyroidism did not show any benefits for the fetus. The American College of Obstetricians and Gynecologists does not recommend routine screening for or treatment of subclinical hypothyroidism during pregnancy.

CASE STUDY #1

Rachel was 28 years old when she became pregnant for the first time. She has had type I diabetes since age 12 and was diagnosed with hypothyroidism at age 22. At that time she started thyroxine replacement, and her TSH was subsequently in the normal range taking 0.150 mg a day. At her first prenatal visit, her TSH level was again in the normal range. TSH was repeated at 16 weeks' gestation, and found to be elevated, so her dose was increased to 0.175 mg daily. Subsequent TSH testing was normal until 32 weeks, when again it was elevated, and her thyroxine dose was increased to 0.200 mg daily, which was continued through the rest of her pregnancy. At term she delivered a normal healthy male infant, who continues to have normal neurologic development at age 5. By six months after delivery, her TSH was again stable on her pre-pregnancy daily dose of 0.150 mg daily.

CASE STUDY #2

Brigit was at 18 weeks' gestation when she complained to her physician of increasing tremor in her hands. She noted this symptom increasing over the past month. Upon questioning, she also described always feeling much warmer than everyone else in the room and excessive sweating. The doctor noted that her pulse was 125 and she appeared to have an enlarged thyroid gland in the front of her neck. The baby's heart rate was not elevated. Laboratory tests were ordered which showed a markedly elevated level of thyroxine and an almost undetectable level of TSH. Methimazole was prescribed along with a beta blocker, and she was asked to return in two weeks. At that time, her pulse was 104 and she described less tremor. Over the next month the TSH and thyroid levels both returned to the normal range, and the beta blocker was discontinued. The methimazole was continued for the rest of the pregnancy, and the fetus never developed tachycardia. Brigit went on to deliver a normal male infant at term, and was referred to an endocrinologist after the pregnancy for further management of her hyperthyroidism.

SUMMARY

Thyroid gland disorders are common among reproductive-age women, and they rarely cause a major problem for pregnancy if they are treated and controlled. Screening for thyroid disease is not indicated unless type I diabetes, a family history of thyroid disease, or symptoms are present. The medications used to treat both hyper- and hypothyroidism are safe to use during pregnancy, and treatment is important if either has been diagnosed. If appropriately treated, problems with the baby are not expected.

CHAPTER 9

AUTOIMMUNE DISORDERS: LUPUS AND ANTIPHOSPHOLIPID ANTIBODIES

THE HUMAN IMMUNE system is a fascinating and complex organization of cells and proteins that evolved to protect us from dangers in the outside world. Its primary function is to recognize dangerous germs and destroy or inactivate them before they cause disease, or at least moderate the disease. Without the immune system we would be at the mercy of every bacterium and virus that exists; with the immune system (and now vaccines and antibiotics) we can fight these invaders in an ever more capable fashion. Some immune cells produce a wide variety of antibodies, proteins that can recognize and bind to different bacteria and viruses, and with the help of other cells, limit the damage until the invaders can be eliminated from the body. We need a well-functioning immune system to survive in a hostile environment of every type of infection.

For reasons still not well understood, sometimes the immune system misidentifies certain molecules in your own body as foreign and begins to attack your own cells. Organs in the body become the target of the immune system, and a self-inflicted disease process begins. Almost any tissue in the body can become a target for this process, including muscles, joints, nerves, blood cells, blood vessels, and membranes, which can lead to complications in almost every organ—brain, peripheral nerves, lungs, thyroid, intestines, pancreas, liver, and kidneys. These complications have a number of different forms, including systemic lupus erythematosus (SLE, or lupus), Sjogren's, scleroderma, Crohn's, type I diabetes, hyper- and hypothyroidism, rheumatoid arthritis, asthma, and multiple sclerosis, to name a few. Sometimes, elements of multiple diseases occur simultaneously, which can be referred to as a mixed connective tissue disorder. All of these conditions share a common cause—the body's immune system produces antibodies against some part of itself, causing inflammation and tissue destruction.

Autoimmune diseases (also referred to as rheumatologic diseases) have become more common over the past few decades, and they affect twice as many women as men. The onset often is during the reproductive years, but some begin later in life. In this chapter, we will review two of these disorders which can significantly affect and complicate pregnancy.

SYSTEMIC LUPUS ERYTHEMATOSUS

Systemic lupus erythematosus, or lupus, is caused by autoantibodies attacking various tissues in the body. The most common of these antibodies are antinuclear antibodies (ANA), and almost all patients with lupus have a positive ANA blood test. However, that is not sufficient to make the diagnosis—at least 4 of the 11 signs or symptoms must be present to make a diagnosis. Some of these criteria include rash, sensitivity to light, mouth ulcers, arthritis, nervous system problems, protein in the urine, and low blood cell counts. Other symptoms could include fatigue, joint or muscle pain, difficulty breathing, and fever. Some people have a mild case, mostly bothered by joint pains and fatigue, while others can have a severe case involving heart and kidney injury. Brain involvement is rare, but is the most feared complication because it can be lethal.

Ninety percent of cases of lupus start in women between the ages of 15 and 44. When this occurs, treatment usually starts with medications that suppress the immune system. Often the first medication is prednisone, a type of steroid to reduce immune system activity. However, continued use of steroids can have many side effects, including high blood pressure, elevated blood sugar, weight gain, bone loss, mood changes, insomnia, and susceptibility to infection. For more severe cases, a stronger immune-suppressing medication may be needed. Ultimately, the goal is disease control with the lowest dose of prednisone possible to reduce the steroid side effects, along with other immune-suppressing agents if needed. Flares of disease activity may occur and medication doses may need to be increased to return the patient to a situation of disease control. Hydroxychloroquine (or Plaquenil) is frequently prescribed to help maintain patients in remission.

As with other autoimmune diseases, maintaining disease control is the highest priority for pregnancy. If you have lupus, the chances of complications during pregnancy are lower if the disease has been well controlled for more than six months prior to conception. Although there are risks associated with taking some immunosuppressive medication during pregnancy, the benefits of disease control outweigh these risks.

RISKS OF LUPUS IN PREGNANCY

Patients with lupus are at increased risk for complications in pregnancy, including miscarriage, poor fetal growth, lupus flares, and development of preeclampsia. These risks are even higher for patients whose disease is not controlled around the time of conception, and also for those patients whose lupus has resulted in hypertension or kidney disease. In addition, there are antibodies found in some patients with lupus that can cross the placenta into the fetus and cause complications. SS-A and SS-B antibodies are present in up to 25% of patients with lupus, and these antibodies can target the fibers in the fetal heart that control heart rate. Disruption of these fibers leads to a slowing of the fetal heart rate (bradycardia) and potentially heart damage (chapter 17). Fortunately, this only occurs in 3% of patients with SS-A or SS-B.

MANAGEMENT OF LUPUS IN PREGNANCY

If you have lupus, planning for pregnancy is important. Discussions with your physician should be centered around getting good disease control for at least six months prior to conception. Medications should be taken that best control the disease and are thought to be compatible with pregnancy. After conception does occur, initial laboratory tests will include baseline kidney function tests and measures of immune disease activity. A test for SS-A and SS-B antibodies should also be performed to determine whether there is risk of the fetus developing bradycardia. If hypertension is present, it should be treated as discussed in chapter 6. The kidney and immune tests are repeated periodically throughout the pregnancy to help assess your disease status, but the SS-A and SS-B tests do not need to be repeated if initially negative. You should also know to report any symptoms to suggest that you might be having a disease flare.

In the second half of pregnancy, it is important that fetal growth be followed with ultrasound to assess for the possibility of growth restriction. Blood pressure should also be monitored closely to watch for signs of preeclampsia development. Beginning sometime in the last two months, assessment of fetal status with either NSTs or BPPs should be performed at least weekly until delivery. If no complications are identified, the pregnancy can be carried to term and a normal outcome for the mother and the baby can be anticipated, but delivery by the due date is often recommended.

ANTIPHOSPHOLIPID ANTIBODY SYNDROME

Antiphospholipid antibodies are autoimmune antibodies that can target various membranes in the body which affect the ability to control clotting. When present, these antibodies have been associated with blood clots forming in both arteries and veins. The antiphospholipid antibodies which have been associated with pregnancy complications are lupus anticoagulant (LAC) and anticardiolipin antibody (ACL). LAC was first identified in patients with prolonged clotting studies, so it was initially thought to be a risk for excessive bleeding. Tests that determine how long it takes for a clot to form are prolonged with LAC, but paradoxically LAC in fact can cause clots to form in various blood vessels of the body. If this occurs in the brain, the result can be a stroke. The presence of LAC was subsequently found in a number of patients with recurrent miscarriage, stillbirths, and severe preeclampsia with only rare normal pregnancies. ACL was then found in the blood of some patients with similar pregnancy complications, with or without LAC also present. Some patients with these antibodies have lupus, but others do not. And most patients with lupus have neither antiphospholipid antibody. Ultimately, the antiphospholipid syndrome (APS) was defined as the presence of one or both of these antibodies in conjunction with either a prior major blood clot or one of the following pregnancy complications: stillbirth, severe preeclampsia before 34 weeks, or three consecutive miscarriages.

In a woman with antiphospholipid antibodies, the prognosis for the pregnancy may depend on why she was tested. If she underwent testing either because of a prior blood clot or because she has lupus, the prognosis is much better than if she was tested because of a prior stillbirth or early severe preeclampsia. With the latter, the recurrence risk is much higher, with some patients having many pregnancies without a successful outcome. In this situation, the fetus can already have significant growth restriction or death by the end of the second trimester, or the patient can develop bleeding or severe preeclampsia before 28 weeks' gestation. This is a very concerning situation which needs to be monitored closely after 20 weeks' gestation.

MANAGEMENT OF ANTIPHOSPHOLIPID SYNDROME

Because this condition is so uncommon, few clinical studies are available to guide management decisions. General consensus has suggested that a patient with APS should be managed based on her medical history. If she has not had one of the severe adverse pregnancy outcomes listed above and no prior blood clots, treatment is not indicated. If she has had a prior blood clot, she should receive blood thinners similar to other patients who have had a prior blood clot (see chapter 12). For those with the syndrome because of a prior adverse pregnancy outcome listed above, most MFM physicians would treat during pregnancy with both blood thinners and low-dose aspirin, beginning by the end of the first trimester. Again, due to lack of data, it is not clear that this treatment will help to prevent another pregnancy complication, but many patients appear to have benefited from this approach.

Because of the risks of poor fetal growth and preeclampsia, women with APS should have periodic ultrasound exams to assess the adequacy of fetal growth. Elevations of the blood pressure or the onset of protein in the urine should generate concern for evolving preeclampsia. If either growth restriction or preeclampsia are present, management should be similar to other situations where these conditions are present. Even if it is not present, many physicians would initiate fetal surveillance with either NSTs or BPPs in the third trimester. If no complications arise, the patient can be delivered at term similar to any other patient without a complication.

OTHER AUTOIMMUNE DISORDERS

Crohn's, Sjogren's, scleroderma, rheumatoid arthritis, and multiple sclerosis are just a few of the many autoimmune disorders that can occur. Some of these cause minimal disruptions to daily life, while others can be quite debilitating. Medications that suppress the immune system can be very helpful in controlling the disease but some, such as steroids, can have significant side effects, as described above. Another medication used for autoimmune disorders is azathioprine, but uncommonly it also can have serious side effects with long-term use.

Most recently a new class of medications has been developed called biologics. Biologics work to block the formation of molecules called cytokines, which cause inflammation. Those biologics developed for treating autoimmune disorders can improve or eliminate symptoms by reducing inflammation. Examples of these include Humera, Remicade, and Embrel. For many patients, treatment with a biologic has provided far better symptom control than was achieved with traditional immune suppressants. And more biologics are coming to market all the time, providing benefits for more and more patients with immune disorders. Most patients do not have side effects, although allergic reactions can occur, and patients may be more susceptible to infections. Other drawbacks include that these medications tend to be very expensive and many need to be given by injection or IV infusion.

Many of the same principles of pregnancy management apply to the other autoimmune disorders as they do to lupus. The disease should be under good control at the time of conception. Testing for SS-A and SS-B antibodies should be performed for patients with Sjogren's syndrome. The risks of developing fetal growth restriction and preeclampsia are not elevated, and fetal surveillance is not routine. Medications used to control the disorder prior to conception are continued during pregnancy, and doses increased or other medications added if disease flares occur. Some concerns have been raised about continuing biologics during pregnancy because of limited safety data. However, a number of these medications have now been used for over a decade with hundreds of women taking them during pregnancy. So far there does not appear to be an increase in miscarriages or fetal malformations with their use; nor does there appear to be any adverse clinical effects on the baby. As such, patients are now often counseled that the benefits of disease control derived from the continuation of biologics during pregnancy outweigh the theoretical risks, and the medications can be continued.

CASE STUDY #1

Tracy had a very bad obstetric history when she presented in the first trimester with her seventh pregnancy. She had suffered three early miscarriages, along with a fetal death in the early second trimester and two stillbirths that had severe growth restriction at the end of the second trimester. She did not have lupus or any other autoimmune disease and no prior episodes of blood clots, but had tested positive for lupus anticoagulant and had a high level of anticardiolipin antibodies. Ultrasound at her first visit showed a normal-appearing embryo, and she was started on shots of the blood thinner enoxaparin (Lovenox) twice a day along with a daily low-dose aspirin tablet. She appeared to be doing well until her 20-week ultrasound showed the fetus about two weeks behind in growth just below the 10th percentile. She was then seen weekly to follow her blood pressure, and the ultrasound was repeated every two weeks. At 24 weeks the fetus was estimated to weigh only 350 grams (12 ounces), and at 26 weeks she was admitted to the hospital because of rising blood pressure and the appearance of protein in her urine. Fetal heart rate monitoring showed some signs of concern, but delivery was delayed in an effort to allow the fetus more time to grow inside the uterus. During the 28th week, Tracy became quite hypertensive despite multiple blood pressure medications, and a decision was made to deliver the fetus by cesarean. The procedure was uncomplicated, but Tracy spent three nights in the ICU postoperatively until her blood pressure was stabilized. The baby weighed 500 grams at birth (1 pound, 2 ounces), and had a prolonged neonatal ICU stay with multiple complications. Nevertheless, after four months he was discharged in good condition, and at five years of age was still developing normally. Tracy recovered to her normal health status and has had no further pregnancies.

CASE STUDY #2

Rashida was 29 years old when she told her rheumatologist that she was interested in getting pregnant. She had been first diagnosed with lupus at age 23, when she developed arthritis in her hands, fatigue, a facial rash, and protein and blood in her urine. She was initially treated with prednisone, but ultimately her lupus was controlled with a combination of mycophenolate and hydroxychloroquine. She had not had any flares in her lupus in over a year. Her rheumatologist told her that she should continue her hydroxychloroquine but stop the mycophenolate in preparation for pregnancy.

At her first prenatal visit, Rashida was feeling well without any change in her symptoms. Her blood pressure was normal as was her kidney function. Testing for antiphospholipid antibodies was negative, but she tested positive for both SS-A and SS-B antibodies. She was told that she would need to come to the office every two weeks starting at 16 weeks to listen to the baby's heart rate to make sure bradycardia was not present. At 26 weeks ultrasound demonstrated that the fetus was growing normally, but at 32 weeks was at the 10th percentile for weight. Weekly NSTs were begun and were reassuring. At 37 weeks, Rashida's blood pressure was now *elevated, and ultrasound showed that the fetus was at the 5th percentile. She was admitted to the hospital for labor induction for suspected preeclampsia with fetal growth restriction. During labor, the fetal heart rate monitoring became non-reassuring, and a decision was made to stop the induction and move to cesarean delivery. The female infant weighed 4½ pounds and had no complications of prematurity. Rashida and the baby were discharged on hospital day three in good condition.*

SUMMARY

Autoimmune disorders are becoming more common among reproductive-age women, and medication is often required to control disease activity. Having the condition well controlled prior to conception reduces the chances of disease flare and complications during pregnancy. The benefits of most medications used to treat these conditions are usually thought to outweigh their risks, and so they are continued throughout the pregnancy to control the disease. Patients with lupus are at increased risk for developing preeclampsia and fetal growth restriction, so more monitoring of these pregnancies is warranted. Patients with the antiphospholipid syndrome and prior adverse pregnancy outcomes, especially those with prior stillbirth or early severe preeclampsia, are at high risk of severe complications, and the prognosis for a successful outcome is guarded. For those patients with other autoimmune disorders the prognosis for a healthy baby without persisting maternal complications is very good.

CHAPTER 10

HEART DISEASE

WHEN MOST PEOPLE think about heart disease, they picture a man over 60 years old, not a woman in her reproductive years. But heart disease is present in all age groups, from infants to senior citizens, and is now the leading cause of death in the United States for women as well as men. There are a number of forms of heart disease, which include cardiac malformations present from birth, problems with the heart valves, arrhythmias, coronary artery disease, and heart muscle malfunction. All of these can be present in a woman during pregnancy and can create challenges for the mother and baby. Some of these heart problems are not significant issues during pregnancy, while others are very concerning and require monitoring and sometimes treatment. For some cardiac problems, such as severe pulmonary hypertension, maternal mortality is a major concern, and termination of pregnancy is often recommended.

By the middle of the first trimester, the mother's heart is already reflecting changes necessary to sustain the pregnancy. Her heart rate has begun to rise, and the amount of blood pumped with each beat increases. Together these result in increased work for the heart to continue to provide oxygen and other nutrients to all of the

Heart Disease 79

mother's organs, and also provide for the needs of the growing uterus and fetus. This workload increases 50% from conception to the end of the second trimester (almost 100% in multiple gestations), and is relatively stable for the remainder of the pregnancy. The hearts of most pregnant women can tolerate this increased workload without difficulty, but for some women the capacity of the heart is overwhelmed, leading to signs of heart failure. If you have heart disease, your cardiologist should work with your obstetrician to assess your level of risk, evaluate your heart function as these changes occur, and treat any signs of cardiac decompensation to keep you safe.

CONGENITAL HEART DISEASE (CHD)

Defects in the formation of the heart are now found in babies more commonly than they were 50 years ago, with the prevalence now being nearly 1% of all births, or about 40,000 each year in the United States.[1] This is most likely due to improved diagnostic techniques identifying more mild types that have less clinical significance. The rate of more serious defects has remained relatively stable over this time period. The types of defects include malformed valves, abnormalities in the vessels leading to and from the heart, and holes in the ventricle walls. For about one in four babies with CHD, the defect is considered critical, meaning that they generally need surgery or other procedures before their first birthday.[2] About 80% of heart defects can be detected by ultrasound by the end of the second trimester.

For those babies with critical defects, surgical techniques have improved so much that most survive into adulthood and lead normal, active lives. However, when a woman born with CHD becomes pregnant, her heart will be stressed more than it has been previously. A general rule of thumb is that the stress of pregnancy is similar to the stress of exercise. If she can exercise vigorously or even walk for a mile at a brisk pace, her heart will most likely tolerate the stress of pregnancy without a problem.

The first step in the evaluation of a patient born with CHD, whether or not it required surgical correction, is an echocardiogram. This is an ultrasound of the heart which can look at flow through the valves and assess how well the heart is pumping blood. If the heart is functioning normally, this test may be repeated later in the pregnancy to be sure that the function remains normal. In this situation, the pregnancy can proceed to term; there is no contraindication to labor and vaginal delivery, and the patient can have an epidural for labor pain. If significant abnormalities are identified on one of the echocardiogram tests, they will be dealt with as described below for the separate issues.

VALVULAR HEART DISEASE

The heart has four valves—two that connect the atria to the ventricles, and two at the outflow of the ventricles (see figure 10.1). The valves are supposed to let blood through during one part of the heart cycle but then close during the second part of the cycle, preventing blood from flowing backwards. Valves can be abnormal either as a congenital defect, or acquired later in life. They can be stenotic, limiting the amount of blood that can go through it, or they can close improperly and have *regurgitation* with blood flowing backwards. Rheumatic fever used to be a major cause of valvular disease in the past, but this is rarely seen in Western countries currently. Concerns relate to which valve is involved and how abnormal the stenosis or regurgitation is. In general, the most concern is for stenosis of the mitral valve (connecting the left atrium to the left ventricle) and stenosis of the aortic valve (connecting the left ventricle to the aorta). Mitral stenosis can be very serious, as the extra fluid of pregnancy that cannot get through the valve backs up into the

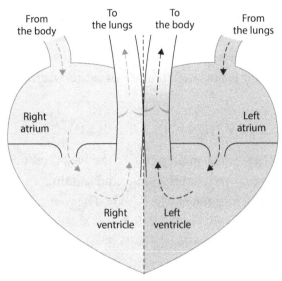

FIGURE 10.1   Schematic of the mother's heart. Blood from the body enters the right atrium (*upper left*), flows through the tricuspid valve, enters the right ventricle, and exits to the lungs through the pulmonic valve, where it releases carbon dioxide and gathers oxygen. Oxygenated blood from the lungs returns to the heart (*upper right*) into the left atrium and passes through the mitral valve into the left ventricle, which then pumps the blood to the body through the aortic valve.

lungs, compromising breathing. If the mitral stenosis is advanced and known prior to the pregnancy, the cardiologist may recommend a procedure to either open up the valve or replace it prior to pregnancy. Aortic valve stenosis can impede the left ventricle's ability to pump sufficient blood into the aorta, resulting in inadequate blood flow to the baby and maternal organs. The stresses of labor will complicate both types of stenosis, and patients with these frequently need cardiac monitoring during labor.

If a woman has had any heart valve replaced, pregnancy is not contraindicated if the valve is working properly. However, those with a mechanical valve will need to continue anticoagulation therapy during the pregnancy so that a blood clot does not form on the valve. Because such a complication is so detrimental, anticoagulation with warfarin (Coumadin) may be recommended in this situation when it is not used in other situations during pregnancy.

LEFT VENTRICULAR DYSFUNCTION

The left ventricle is the main pump of the heart, taking blood that has picked up oxygen from the lungs and sending it to the aorta to be distributed all over the mother's body. The ventricle pumps blood through the aortic valve in the first half of the heart cycle (systole), and fills with blood through the mitral valve in the second half of the cycle (diastole). Normally in the first half of the cycle, the left ventricle sends 50–60% of the blood it contains through the aortic valve (the ejection fraction, or EF). But there are situations where it pumps less than 50% due to injury of the heart muscle itself. Things that can cause this include a prior heart attack, damage to the muscle from a prior infection, and some genetic conditions where the heart muscle weakens over time, also known as hereditary cardiomyopathy. With reduced ejection fraction, the ventricle may not be able to meet the excess demands of pregnancy, resulting in heart failure. Activity may need to be limited to reduce demands on the heart.

If a woman with left ventricular dysfunction becomes pregnant, echocardiograms may need to be performed periodically to look for signs of further reductions in the left ventricular ejection fraction. Medications may be added to strengthen the contractions of the heart muscle, and a diuretic (medication that increases elimination of water from the body) may be helpful in preventing fluid from backing up into the lungs. For patients with markedly reduced ejection fraction, the pregnancy may need to be delivered early to prevent the situation from deteriorating further. Labor does increase the demands on the heart, but this can be eased with epidural anesthesia, and is still often safer for the mother than the stresses associated with cesarean delivery.

PERIPARTUM CARDIOMYOPATHY

There are some women with no prior heart disease who experience a complication known as peripartum cardiomyopathy (PPCM). This is defined as a significant drop in left ventricular output in the last month of pregnancy or the five months after delivery. It was first referred to as postpartum cardiomyopathy as most cases occur after delivery, but it is now referred to as peripartum cardiomyopathy in recognition that in some patients it develops prior to delivery. Some of the risk factors for PPCM include obesity, twins, advanced maternal age, and preeclampsia. These patients frequently present with swelling and shortness of breath, and clinical findings include fluid in the lungs. The severity depends on how low the ejection fraction drops—the lower the EF, the more severe the condition. Immediate treatment may include administering oxygen, diuretic medications (to eliminate fluid), and medications to strengthen heart muscle contractions. For most women, heart function returns to normal over weeks to months, but for some the damage is permanent and a heart transplant may be lifesaving.

If cardiac function returns to normal with a normal ejection fraction and a normal stress test, having another pregnancy may be an option. However, the recurrence risk is 30%, and there is no way to predict which women will have a recurrence. For those women whose heart function does not return to normal, another pregnancy is routinely discouraged.

PULMONARY HYPERTENSION

Pulmonary hypertension occurs when the blood is flowing from the right ventricle through the lungs at a higher pressure than normal.

This can occur spontaneously, known as primary pulmonary hypertension, or as a result of having another condition which stresses the heart. These conditions include lung disease, left ventricular dysfunction, prior pulmonary embolisms, and a defect in the wall (septum) separating the sides of the heart. Patients with pulmonary hypertension often have symptoms of shortness of breath, chest pain, and lightheadedness. There are medications that can help reduce the elevated pressure, but there is no cure. For those women with significant limitation of activity due to pulmonary hypertension, the risk of death during pregnancy is substantial and pregnancy is routinely discouraged. If maternal pulmonary hypertension is identified before the third trimester, termination of pregnancy can be lifesaving.

CASE STUDY #1

LaRhonda was doing well through the first two trimesters of her third pregnancy, but she then began to experience shortness of breath, lethargy with walking short distances, and swelling in her legs up to her knees. When breathing became too difficult, she went to the emergency room and was found to have a rapid pulse and was breathing 32 times a minute at rest. A chest X-ray showed significant fluid in her lungs and an enlarged heart. An echocardiogram showed decreased contractility of her left ventricle and an EF of 35%, with thickening of the heart walls. There was a strong family history of heart disease, but she was not aware of any diagnosis. She was started on oxygen therapy, given multiple doses of a diuretic medication, and was started on a beta blocker and digoxin to strengthen her heart's contractions. She was admitted to the hospital and over the next two days her breathing improved while she passed a large amount of urine. After discharge, she limited her activity and continued her medications. Her symptoms were still well controlled, but repeat echocardiograms continued to show a decrease in her EF of 30–40%. She was followed closely by a cardiologist and her maternal-fetal medicine specialist, and the fetus was growing normally. By the end of the third trimester, the increasing demands of the pregnancy on her heart resulted in worsening of symptoms, but her oxygen levels remained satisfactory with minimal exertion. A decision was made to induce her labor at 37 weeks, and epidural anesthesia was given for pain control and to reduce her cardiac workload during labor. After a six-hour labor, she delivered a 6-pound, 5-ounce baby girl in good condition. LaRhonda was monitored over the next 48 hours in the ICU, and her symptoms improved as she passed more urine. After discharge on day four after delivery, she improved symptomatically over the next few months, but six months later her ejection fraction was still less than 40%. Genetic testing confirmed that she had an inherited hypertrophic cardiomyopathy. It was suggested that she tell other family members that they should have genetic testing to see if they had the same condition, and her baby should be tested as well. LaRhonda was advised that any future pregnancy could be similarly complicated, and that she should have regular checkups with a cardiologist to monitor her condition. If her ejection fraction dropped in the future, she might need a heart transplant.

CASE STUDY #2

When she was a teenager, Ariana developed a severe staph infection which spread through her blood to her heart. Her mitral valve was damaged by the infection, resulting in mitral stenosis. She recovered from the infection after a long course of antibiotics, and her mitral stenosis was judged to be mild. She was no longer able to exercise vigorously, but otherwise was able to do most other activities, and was no longer followed by a cardiologist. When she became pregnant at the age of 23, an echocardiogram showed that *the mitral valve had moderate stenosis, but she was still asymptomatic. She was referred to a cardiologist to follow her closely during the pregnancy. At 28 weeks, Ariana began to notice more fatigue and shortness of breath when walking more than short distances. A diuretic was started and it was recommended that she limit her activity. At 32 weeks, it was noted that her heart rate was now elevated and a beta blocker was added to the diuretic. When breathing became more difficult at 37 weeks, delivery was recommended. Epidural anesthesia was given prior to starting the induction, and the amount of IV fluids given was limited. When she became completely dilated, she was instructed not to push (the effort would excessively strain her heart), and the baby's head was allowed to spontaneously descend low in the pelvis, allowing for a safe forceps delivery. A 6-pound baby girl was delivered in good condition. Ariana was transferred to the ICU for 24 hours of monitoring, and then discharged with her daughter on postpartum day three. Six months later, a procedure was performed to relieve the stenosis of the mitral valve.*

SUMMARY

How a woman with a heart disorder will do during pregnancy depends on the condition and its severity. Women with many of these conditions do very well during pregnancy, but there are some conditions where pregnancy is a big risk. A general rule is that those women who can exercise moderately will tolerate the stresses of pregnancy. But all women with heart disorders should discuss pregnancy with their cardiologist before conception, and tests such as an echocardiogram or cardiac stress test can be helpful in elucidating the prognosis.

CHAPTER 11

KIDNEY DISEASE

THE KIDNEYS SERVE an important role in filtering waste products from the body and maintaining normal levels of water and minerals. They also stimulate the bone marrow to make blood cells and eliminate medications and toxins. During pregnancy, the workload of the kidneys increases approximately 50% as measured by how much blood is filtered by the kidneys per minute. The best measure of how well the kidneys are functioning is the blood level of creatinine, a waste product of digestion of protein and the normal breakdown of muscle tissue. Creatinine levels vary among individuals, but most people with normal kidney function have blood levels between 0.7 and 1.3 mg/dL. In pregnancy, creatinine levels are routinely between 0.5 and 0.7 mg/dL because of the increased filtration present after the first trimester. Elevations of the creatinine level above normal are a sign of kidney disease, as is the finding of blood or protein in the urine. Most people with kidney disease are asymptomatic until the disease has progressed to an advanced stage.

TYPES OF KIDNEY DISEASE

Kidney disease, also called renal disease, is often divided into acute and chronic illnesses. Other than kidney infections, kidney disease that arises during pregnancy is extremely uncommon. Chronic diseases can be present at birth (examples include childhood polycystic kidney disease and absence of a kidney) or arise during one's lifetime. These can be immune related (such as lupus nephritis), genetic, or due to another condition (hypertension, diabetes), or they can arise on their own. Treatments vary by the type of disease, and medications used include steroids, immunosuppressives, diuretics, and ACE inhibitors which block certain enzymes. With long-standing kidney disease, many patients develop hypertension, which needs to be treated.

RISKS ASSOCIATED WITH KIDNEY DISEASE AND PREGNANCY

With renal disease, pregnancy has a higher risk of preterm labor, fetal growth restriction, stillbirth, and development of preeclampsia. The level of increased risk correlates with the stage of the disease, and the maternal blood creatinine level is the best determinant of disease stage. As stated previously, the creatinine level decreases in normal pregnancy, so levels above 0.7 mg/dL indicate some degree of compromised kidney function. Creatinine levels of 1.4 mg/dL or higher before pregnancy have been reported to have preterm delivery rates of 60%, fetal growth restriction rates of nearly 40%, fetal death rates of 7%, and preeclampsia rates of 50%.[1] Further, up to 50% of women with elevated creatinine levels see these values rise further during pregnancy, indicating some degree of deterioration in renal function. For most, the kidney function returns to baseline after pregnancy, but a significant portion of women starting with a creatinine level of 2 mg/dL or higher have worse kidney function after pregnancy than before. Some women with the highest creatinine levels progress to kidney failure, and will need dialysis or a kidney transplant.

MANAGEMENT OF PREGNANCIES WITH KIDNEY DISEASE

The focus of pregnancy management starts with following kidney function. If creatinine levels begin to rise or protein levels in the urine increase, the dosage of medication used to treat the kidney disease may need to be increased. Elevations in blood pressure should be treated with the medications as discussed in chapter 6. In the second half of pregnancy, ultrasound is used to assess fetal growth. Fetal surveillance should begin in the third trimester, earlier if preeclampsia or fetal growth restriction has been diagnosed. Unless indicated sooner, delivery is routinely performed before the patient's due date.

In the third trimester, it is often difficult to distinguish worsening renal disease from evolving preeclampsia. Both can have elevation in blood pressure and an increase in protein in the urine, along with rising creatinine levels. Medication can be used to control the blood pressure, but worsening status may necessitate a move to delivery.

PREGNANCY IN PATIENTS WITH RENAL TRANSPLANTS

After successful kidney transplantation, renal function often returns to normal with creatinine levels at or below 1.0 mg/dL. It is usually recommended that patients wait at least one year after they receive a new kidney before attempting pregnancy. Medications taken to prevent rejection may need to be changed to ones more compatible with pregnancy, and this is usually recommended before conception. During the pregnancy it is important to check creatinine levels periodically, as well as anti-rejection drug levels to make sure they stay in the recommended range. Rising creatinine levels or protein in the urine can be a sign of rejection, which should be treated aggressively. But in a patient with a transplanted kidney which is functioning well and with no hypertension present, the prognosis for a successful pregnancy is very good.

PREGNANCY WITH A SINGLE KIDNEY

Some people are born with only one kidney, while others may have only one because they have donated the other one or had one removed due to disease. If the single kidney is functioning normally and the serum creatinine level is normal, these patients routinely do well during pregnancy. Nonetheless, those women with only one kidney should discuss this with their doctors prior to pregnancy, when possible.

CASE STUDY #1

Juana had long-standing kidney disease due to type I diabetes. When she conceived, she had a blood creatinine level of 2.5 mg/dL and her urine had 3+ protein. At her first visit she was counseled that her risk of adverse pregnancy outcome was quite high, and that her kidney function could deteriorate to kidney failure during the pregnancy. Her blood sugars were brought under good control, and her hypertension was controlled with a beta blocker. By 20 weeks her creatinine had risen to 3.5 with 4+ protein in her urine. Ultrasound showed a normally developing fetus at the 20th percentile for growth. By 26 weeks, the fetus was now below the 10th percentile, and weekly fetal surveillance was begun with NSTs. At 30 weeks she was hospitalized for blood pressure control and a second medication was added to the beta blocker. At 32 weeks a decision was made to proceed with delivery, as her blood pressure was increasingly difficult to control and superimposed preeclampsia was likely. A female infant was delivered by cesarean weighing 2½ pounds, and she was discharged from the neonatal ICU at six weeks of age weighing 5 pounds. Juana recovered satisfactorily from the surgery, but her kidney function continued to deteriorate. Two months after delivery she was started on dialysis and placed on the transplant list.

Three years later she presented again pregnant, having received a kidney and pancreas transplant the year before. Her diabetes resolved with the new pancreas, and her new kidney was functioning well. At the first visit, her creatinine level was 0.8 mg/dL, there was no protein in her urine, and her blood pressure was normal on no medications. Her pregnancy progressed without complication, with the fetus growing normally and her creatinine level staying below 1.0 mg/dL. At 39 weeks, she underwent a repeat cesarean without complication, delivering a boy weighing 6½ pounds who did well. Both she and the baby were discharged on day four, and her transplanted kidney continued to function normally.

CASE STUDY #2

Betty was known to have autosomal dominant polycystic kidney disease (ADPKD), a condition where a large number of cysts form in both kidneys. Her father has this condition, as do two of four brothers. Betty was first diagnosed with this condition at the age of 22, when an ultrasound showed the presence of characteristic cysts in her kidneys. She was now 28 years old and came for an MFM consultation to discuss the possibility of getting pregnant. She was diagnosed with hypertension four years previously, which was currently well controlled with an ACE inhibitor. Tests were ordered which included a serum creatinine of 1.4, and an ultrasound showed no progression of the cysts in her kidneys, and no cysts in her liver. Counseling included discussing the increased risks of preterm labor, fetal growth restriction, stillbirth, and development of preeclampsia, as well as a 50% chance of passing the condition to each child.

When Betty became pregnant, her blood pressure medication was switched to nifedipine, which controlled her hypertension well. Daily low-dose aspirin was recommended beginning at the end of the first trimester. She did well during the pregnancy, with a drop in her creatinine level, which was sustained throughout the pregnancy, and repeat ultrasounds continued to show that the fetus was growing normally. Weekly NSTs were initiated at 32 weeks and were reassuring. However, at 38 weeks she was diagnosed with preeclampsia, and labor induction was initiated. After a 20-hour labor, she delivered a healthy female infant weighing 7 pounds. After delivery, the ACE inhibitor was restarted for blood pressure control, and at her six-week checkup, her serum creatinine was back to her pre-pregnancy level.

SUMMARY

Women with kidney disease routinely do well during pregnancy if the blood creatinine level is in or near the normal range. Even so, the risk of preterm delivery, preeclampsia, and fetal growth restriction is increased relative to women without kidney disease. These risks are even higher, with elevations in the blood creatinine level, and there is some risk that kidney function can deteriorate permanently with pregnancy. Kidney function as well as fetal growth need to be monitored during the pregnancy, but patients will likely deliver at term if these remain normal and preeclampsia does not develop. Women with transplanted kidneys also have a good prognosis if the kidney is functioning well at the beginning of the pregnancy.

CHAPTER 12

BLOOD CLOTS: PULMONARY EMBOLISM AND DEEP VEIN THROMBOSIS

THE CIRCULATORY SYSTEM has the ability to maintain blood flowing through the arteries and veins without clotting, but then to form clots to stop bleeding when blood escapes through lacerations or injury. The mechanisms that stop bleeding from lacerations and those that prevent clots from forming in major blood vessels are complex but important for the proper balance of these two functions. In pregnancy, the balance is tipped toward coagulation, presumably to help prevent excess bleeding at the time of delivery. But this also means that when pregnant, and for six weeks after, women are at increased risk of forming blood clots in major veins in the legs, blood vessels in the brain (strokes), and blood vessels in the lungs.

In 2010 Serena Williams was sidelined from tennis for an extended period by a blood clot in her lungs. Having had a pulmonary embolism put her at increased risk for a recurrence at any time for the rest of her life. And indeed, that is what happened soon after she delivered her daughter in 2017, a situation which she referred to as life threatening.[1] In fact, pregnant women are four times more likely to have a clotting problem than nonpregnant women, and this risk continues for at least six weeks after delivery.[2] African American women are at even higher risk than White women, and this contributes significantly to the disparity in maternal mortality between races. It is of particular importance that all women inform their obstetric provider of any risk factors for thrombosis in pregnancy. Factors that increase the risk of forming a clot in a vein (or venous thrombosis) include having had a clot in a prior pregnancy, having a close relative with a prior thrombosis, air travel, surgery, and the presence of antiphospholipid antibodies or a clotting gene abnormality.

Blood clots that form in superficial veins of the body can be painful but do not usually raise serious concerns. Blood clots that form in the deep veins (deep venous thrombosis, or DVT) are of more concern, as portions of the clot can break off and travel back up the veins to the heart and then into the lungs. A clot that travels to the lungs is referred to as a pulmonary embolism (PE), but clots can also form in the lungs spontaneously without having come from a clot in the legs. Most DVTs and PEs resolve without having long-term effects, but some PEs can be life threatening and need to be taken seriously. Symptoms of leg DVTs include swelling, pain, and redness; symptoms of PEs include chest pain, difficulty breathing, rapid breathing rate, and rapid heart rate. The diagnosis of a DVT is made with an ultrasound of the affected limb, while a PE is diagnosed with a CT scan of the chest. Strokes caused by blood clots in brain blood vessels are diagnosed with either a CT scan or MRI.

DVT AND PE IN PREGNANCY

Because of the increased risk of DVT and PE in pregnancy, patients and their providers should have an elevated level of suspicion when symptoms arise. Concerns should be evaluated promptly so that treatment can be started quickly should a clot be identified. This is usually performed in an emergency department, where resources for ultrasound and CT scans are usually available in a short period of time. Ultrasound does not involve any radiation, and a CT scan has a very low level of radiation exposure for the fetus. The importance of identifying a PE if present outweighs this level of radiation risk. There are other tests for PE available, but they are not nearly as accurate as a CT scan.

If a DVT or PE is identified, a blood thinner is prescribed, usually a low molecular weight heparin (LMWH) such as enoxaparin (Lovenox). This medication is administered by injection, and usually is given more than once a day because it is metabolized more rapidly during pregnancy. Blood levels assessing a clotting factor (anti-Xa) drawn four hours after a dose are used to ensure adequate anticoagulation, with dose adjustments as necessary. Heparin does not cross the placenta, so there is no effect on the fetus. There are other injectable blood thinners that are usually given only once a day, but these are less well studied in pregnancy. Oral blood thinners are rarely used during pregnancy because they can cross into the bloodstream of the fetus and result in fetal bleeding. The LMWH is continued for the remainder of the pregnancy and six weeks after delivery, when the risk of clotting due to pregnancy has returned to a nonpregnant level of risk. However, it may be recommended that anticoagulation be continued until six to nine months after the clot was diagnosed. Anticoagulation is usually stopped for labor and delivery, and restarted when it is thought that the risk of excess bleeding is minimal.

Some patients develop thromboses related to an inherited genetic mutation they carry. One such mutation is known as Factor V Leiden; another is a mutation of clotting factor II, also known as the prothrombin mutation. A rarer mutation leads to antithrombin III deficiency. The presence of antiphospholipid antibodies (chapter 9) also increases the risk of thrombosis. Patients who develop a DVT or PE should be tested for these abnormalities, known as thrombophilias, as the finding of any of these will likely influence treatment decisions in the future.

MANAGEMENT OF PATIENTS AT INCREASED RISK FOR THROMBOSIS

Treatment recommendations for those at increased risk are based on consensus because studies have not been performed to determine optimal dosing in each situation. If a woman enters pregnancy with a known risk factor for thrombosis, treatment decisions will be based on her level of risk. If she has had a prior thrombosis, either a DVT or PE, she is given LMWH. However, this is usually once-a-day injections without need for checking anti-Xa levels (low dose or prophylactic dosing). The same approach can be used for patients with a thrombophilia and a close relative with a prior thrombotic episode. Women at higher risk are often treated with an adjusted-dose approach with twice-daily injections, trying to achieve higher levels of anti-Xa. Higher risk is conveyed by having had two or more prior thromboses, or a prior thrombosis with multiple thrombophilias. For these patients, the risk of thrombosis begins to increase in the first trimester, but treatment with LMWH can wait for both an ultrasound that confirms a viable pregnancy and cessation of any bleeding that may occur. Treatment continues until six weeks after delivery.

CASE STUDY #1

Jenae came for her first obstetric appointment at eight weeks' gestation, and ultrasound showed a normal singleton fetus. She reported having had some bleeding two weeks before, but was now only spotting. Four years previously she was diagnosed with a pulmonary embolism while taking birth control pills and was treated with warfarin pills for nine months without complications. Two years later she had a DVT in her left thigh and was again treated for nine months with warfarin. Testing revealed that she had a single gene for Factor V Leiden, but no history of thrombosis in any close relative. Because of her having two prior thromboses and the thrombophilia, the decision was made to treat her with adjusted-dose enoxaparin during the pregnancy, although it was not started until 10 weeks, when her spotting had ceased for seven days. The enoxaparin dose was based on her weight (1 mg enoxaparin for each kilogram of body weight, rounded to the nearest 10 mg) every 12 hours, and a week later her anti-Xa level drawn four hours after a dose was in the desired range.

Jenae's pregnancy continued uncomplicated, and her anti-Xa level was repeated at 20 weeks of gestation. The level was below the desired range, so her dose of enoxaparin was increased by 10 mg. It was increased again at 32 weeks, when her level was again low, and a repeat anti-Xa level was then appropriate. A decision was made to induce her labor at 39 weeks to be able to plan for the delivery. She took her last dose of enoxaparin the morning before the induction, so that she was 24 hours past her last dose when the induction was started. Patients are not eligible for epidural anesthesia until 24 hours past the last injection of adjusted-dose enoxaparin to avoid the risk of the needle causing bleeding near the spinal cord while anticoagulated. Jenae was able to receive an epidural at her request six hours into the induction, and 12 hours later delivered a healthy baby boy vaginally without excess bleeding. The enoxaparin was restarted 12 hours after delivery and continued for six weeks.

CASE STUDY #2

At Teresa's first prenatal visit at 10 weeks of gestation, she told her physician that she had been diagnosed with a DVT eight years previously while she was taking birth control pills. She had no other medical issues or prior thromboses, and no close relatives who had experienced blood clots. Testing for thrombophilias revealed that she carried the prothrombin mutation. She was started on *low-dose Lovenox injections once a day, and anti-Xa levels were not recommended. She did well until 22 weeks, when she called the physician's office to report the onset of pain in her right leg associated with redness and swelling. She was instructed to come to the emergency room, where an ultrasound showed a large clot in her femoral vein above the knee. She was switched to adjusted-dose Lovenox injections twice a day, and factor Xa levels were checked to make sure they remained at the appropriate level. At 39 weeks, she took her last injection in the morning, with induction scheduled 24 hours later. She was able to receive an epidural for anesthesia, but her labor stalled out at 8 cm and a cesarean delivery was performed. Twelve hours after the surgery, her Lovenox was restarted after it was confirmed that her bleeding was minimal, and continued for another five months.*

SUMMARY

Women are at increased risk for forming blood clots in their veins and lungs during pregnancy, and those with other risk factors are at even higher risk. These blood clots could potentially lead to serious consequences for the mother, and symptoms suggesting a clot should be investigated promptly. If a venous thrombosis is identified during pregnancy, testing for a thrombophilia should be performed and anticoagulation initiated. For those at increased risk for a thrombosis during pregnancy a prophylactic dose of enoxaparin is used except for those at even higher risk. With this approach to treatment, the patient will be well protected from having another thrombotic event and a normal pregnancy outcome can be expected.

CHAPTER 13

UTERINE ANOMALIES AND FIBROIDS

A NORMAL ADULT uterus is the size of your fist, and serves little function other than carrying a pregnancy. It consists of a muscular body with the fallopian tubes connected to each side at the top, and a cervix at the bottom (see figure 13.1). There is an inner layer called the endometrium, a thick muscular layer known as the myometrium, and a thin outer layer of tissue, which is the serosa.

The uterus forms long before birth and remains relatively small until puberty. It is not normally examined by a health care provider in childhood, so abnormalities of uterine development are rarely identified until adulthood. Even then, most abnormalities are asymptomatic and undetected. Yet up to 5% of women are born with a malformation in their uterus. Most of these are minor aberrations and do not affect the ability to conceive and carry a pregnancy. When evaluating patients having trouble conceiving and carrying to term, 5–10% are found to have an abnormality possibly playing a role.[1]

Uterine fibroids (also called myomas or leiomyomas) are benign muscle tumors that grow in the uterus. Some studies report that fibroids can be found in more than half of women of European ancestry and are even more common in African American women. Some women have a single fibroid, while others have many. Most

Female Reproductive System

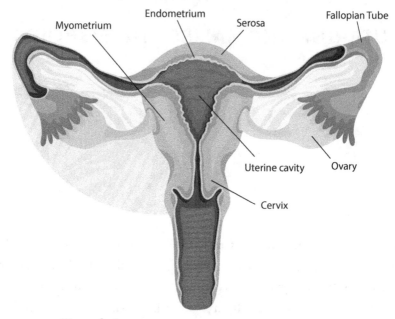

FIGURE 13.1 Normal uterus.
Source: Courtesy of nmfotograf, iStock.

are asymptomatic, although some can cause excess menstrual bleeding and anemia. All but the smallest fibroids can usually be seen on ultrasound, so they are frequently first identified when a woman has her first ultrasound during pregnancy.

TYPES OF UTERINE ANOMALIES AND COMPLICATIONS

Of the many types of uterine anomalies, bicornuate, didelphys, unicornuate, and septate uterus are the most common. These can be differentiated in a number of ways, but the most common method now is MRI. A bicornuate uterus has an indentation in the dome which divides the uterine cavity into two sides. A uterus didelphys, or double uterus, can look like a bicornuate uterus from the outside but has two separate uterine cavities, which sometimes connect to separate cervices. These two cervices can be seen on pelvic examination and can have a septum (flap of tissue) between them extending down the vagina. A unicornuate uterus is similar to a uterus didelphys but has only one of the sides, or horns. A septate uterus looks normal from the outside but has a thin wall of tissue coming down from the top of variable length (see figure 13.2).

All of these uterine anomalies increase the chance of miscarriage, preterm birth, and the baby not being head down at the time of labor, but to different degrees. Unicornuate uterus and uterus didelphys have the highest risk of preterm birth, while septate uterus has the highest risk of miscarriage. Uterine anomalies can be a cause of infertility but are not a risk to the mother once she is pregnant. All of these anomalies have been associated with fetal growth

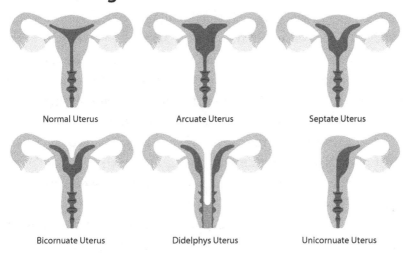

FIGURE 13.2 Types of uterine anomalies.
Source: Courtesy of Guzaliia Filimonova, iStock.

restriction, and the percentage of fetuses that are breech or transverse at term may be as high as 40%.[2]

MANAGEMENT OF UTERINE ANOMALIES

If you are known to have a uterine anomaly, your pregnancy management will not change. Signs and symptoms of preterm labor should be evaluated, and fetal growth should be monitored. Once the patient is in the last month of pregnancy, the fetal presentation should be assessed to determine whether the head is down. Otherwise, pregnancy care is routine. For the patient with multiple miscarriages or preterm deliveries, the uterus should be evaluated to determine if an anomaly is present. If there is a uterine septum, removal of the septum using a hysteroscope (fiberoptic instrument inserted through the cervix) may improve the chances of a successful pregnancy.

UTERINE FIBROIDS

Fibroids are classified by their location in the uterus. Submucosal fibroids are situated under the endometrium and protrude into the uterine cavity, where the fetus grows. Intramural fibroids are embedded in the muscular wall of the uterus, and subserosal fibroids lie between the muscular layer and the outer serosal covering of the uterus. A pedunculated fibroid grows on a stalk, either into the uterine cavity or away from the outside of the uterus. As noted previously, most fibroids are asymptomatic, and most women with fibroids do not know they have them. A woman can have a single fibroid or multiple ones in different locations and of varying sizes. Fibroids can interfere with the ability to get pregnant, and the issues they cause in pregnancy depend on their size and location (see figure 13.3).

A first-trimester ultrasound may note one or more fibroids in the uterus, but no action is necessary at this time. Some fibroids grow in

Uterine Fibroids

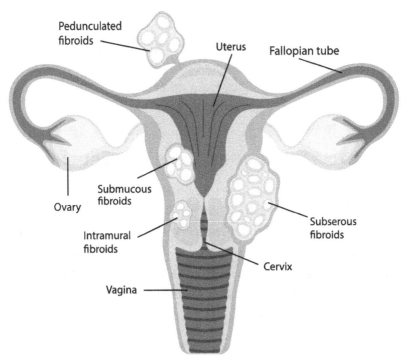

FIGURE 13.3   Different types of fibroids by location.
Source: Courtesy of Kristina Bulgakova, iStock.

the first half of pregnancy due to the influence of the pregnancy's estrogen production. If the growth is too rapid, the fibroid can outgrow its blood supply. When this happens, the muscle cells in the fibroid die, or infarct, which can result in significant pain. But this fibroid infarction rarely causes problems for the pregnancy, and the pain usually resolves within 1–2 weeks. Pain medication is often helpful in getting the patient through this period until the pain resolves.

Subserosal fibroids rarely cause a problem during the pregnancy, even if they grow. Most women with intramural fibroids have normal pregnancies, but some studies show an increased risk of preterm birth and breech or transverse presentation at delivery, especially if the fibroid is large.[3] If the placenta implants over the fibroid, there is an increased risk of placental abruption. Submucosal fibroids are associated with increased risks of difficulty conceiving and miscarriage. And a fibroid located in the lower part of the uterus can block the baby from descending in the vagina during labor, making a cesarean delivery necessary.

MANAGEMENT OF FIBROIDS IN PREGNANCY

In general, the finding of uterine fibroids in pregnancy does not warrant any intervention, as most fibroids do not interfere with pregnancy progress. If a patient has difficulty conceiving or has a miscarriage thought to be related to a submucosal fibroid, removal of this fibroid may be performed with a hysteroscope before the patient attempts to conceive again. Otherwise, fibroids are best left alone unless they are causing other health problems.

CASE STUDY #1

Loretta came for her first prenatal visit at nine weeks' gestation. An ultrasound revealed a 5-centimeter intramural fibroid at the top of her uterus. She had no complaints regarding pain in this area. She did well until 19 weeks, when she came to the office complaining of moderately severe pain in her lower abdomen. An ultrasound now showed that the fibroid had grown to 11 centimeters in diameter with signs of degeneration suggesting that it had outgrown its blood supply. The fetus was growing normally. Loretta was given pain medication and reassured. Two weeks later she reported that the pain had now resolved. The rest of the pregnancy was uncomplicated, and she delivered a healthy boy at 40 weeks weighing 8 pounds, 2 ounces.

CASE STUDY #2

After Mary Kate's second first-trimester miscarriage, her physician discussed the option of evaluating her for a uterine anomaly with MRI. With this imaging, her uterus was noted to be normally shaped but appeared to have a septum descending down from the top of the uterus. A hysteroscopy was recommended to remove it, and a scope was inserted through her cervix, allowing visualization of the uterine cavity. A uterine septum was seen extending down 5 centimeters, essentially dividing the uterine cavity in two. The septum was removed by hysteroscope without complication. Two months later, Mary Kate conceived a twin gestation. This pregnancy was complicated by the development of premature rupture of membranes at 32 weeks, for which she was hospitalized for close observation. At 33 weeks, she developed preeclampsia and labor was induced. She delivered a male and a female infant vaginally, and both were discharged in good condition after a three-week stay in the neonatal ICU.

SUMMARY

The prognosis for patients with either a uterine anomaly or fibroids is generally good. Some types of anomalies as well as submucosal fibroids increase the chances of miscarriage, while other types of anomalies and intramural fibroids increase the chances of preterm delivery. Management of pregnancies with either uterine anomalies or fibroids is routine unless symptoms develop.

CHAPTER 14

CANCER AND PREGNANCY

FORTUNATELY, a cancer diagnosis made during pregnancy is rare, although 7.5% of all cancers are diagnosed between the ages of 20 and 44,[1] and some form of cancer occurs in 1 of every 1,000 pregnancies. Breast cancer is the most common malignancy identified, occurring once in every 3,000 pregnancies.[2] Other types of cancer identified on occasion during pregnancy include colon, lung, cervical, ovarian, and leukemia. A cancer diagnosis is always a shock, especially in someone young. Being pregnant at the time of diagnosis makes the situation much more complicated to diagnose and manage.

These days, most cancers have a good chance of remission or cure if caught at an early stage. The things that determine the prognosis are the type of cancer, at what stage it is diagnosed, and whether there is evidence of spread from the primary tumor. Although the normal immune suppression and hormonal changes of pregnancy could theoretically accelerate the growth and spread of cancer, there is no evidence that this happens. The test to determine the type of cancer is most often a biopsy. Staging and spread are usually assessed with radiologic tests, including X-rays, CT scanning, and MRI. While X-rays and CT scans involve some radiation exposure, it is usually a low level of radiation, and the information gained is vital to planning for management. Treatment may involve surgery, chemotherapy, high-dose radiation, or a combination of these.

MANAGEMENT OF CANCER IN PREGNANCY

The first discussion for a patient with a new diagnosis of cancer should be with a cancer specialist, or oncologist. Many oncologists now specialize in a particular type of cancer, so referral should be made to a physician with expertise with the type of cancer found. The physician will assess the available information from the tests that have been performed and determine whether further testing would be helpful for management decisions. Once the needed information is available, the oncologist should recommend a type of treatment and explain why this is the best approach. She should also give the patient the prognosis for recovery from the cancer. This could be a likelihood for a complete cure or remission, or chances of survival for a given period of time (e.g., chances for survival for five years). Additionally, the patient should learn what the treatment schedule should be and how soon it should start.

With this information, the pregnant patient should then be seen by a maternal-fetal medicine specialist. The first job for this specialist is to emphasize that the health of the mother always comes first. Her prognosis should in no way be compromised for concerns about the effect of treatment on the fetus, though of course those concerns will often be paramount for the expectant mother. She should receive the therapy which gives her the best chance to beat this terrible disease. Most biopsies and many surgeries not in the abdomen can be performed without an adverse effect on the fetus, and anesthesia is generally not thought to be a problem during pregnancy. Chemotherapy can have significant side effects for the mother, including fatigue, hair loss, anemia, mouth sores, nausea, and vomiting. But surprisingly, most chemotherapy medications seem to be well tolerated by a fetus when administered in the second and third trimesters.[3] This may be because some of the chemotherapy is modified or filtered by the placenta so that the drug concentration in the fetal circulation is thought to be significantly less than in the maternal circulation. A small number of chemotherapy agents are thought to be toxic to the fetus;[4] there are often other agents that can be used instead without adversely affecting the mother's prognosis.

There is ample evidence over the past few decades where chemotherapy is given during the second and third trimester without causing birth defects or harm to the fetus. Preterm delivery is more common, and there is a small increase in the percentage of babies born with growth restriction, but it is not clear whether this is an effect of the chemotherapy or the underlying cancer. After delivery, babies may have a transient reduction in some cells of the immune system, but this does not appear to affect the function of their immune system or other systems.[5] And follow-up studies have shown chemotherapy exposure after the first trimester has no effect on later cognitive ability, school performance, or behavioral competence.[6] For these reasons, patients should be reassured that full treatment for their cancer can be pursued even if they are pregnant, without a significant effect on their fetus. And the prognosis for remission and survival is not worse because of being pregnant.

There are occasions where radiation therapy is recommended during pregnancy, either by itself or in addition to chemotherapy and/or surgery. This is only undertaken if radiation treatment will improve the patient's prognosis and cannot wait until after the pregnancy. High doses of radiation to the fetus used for cancer therapy can cause miscarriage or stillbirth, brain injury, slowing of fetal growth, and increased chances of developing cancer later in childhood. There are some strategies to reduce the amount of radiation that the fetus is exposed to, but inevitably the fetus will have some exposure, as the treatment cannot be completely focused only on the tumor. Fortunately, the need for radiation treatment for cancer during pregnancy is very uncommon.

Of course, every expectant mother will have her own concerns and every case is different, so exploring options with a health care team with experience in treating pregnant women for cancer is essential. It is uncommon that termination of the pregnancy will improve the mother's prognosis, unless the optimal treatment is not possible with a fetus present. An example of this might be abdominal radiation for lymphoma, in which case termination of pregnancy may be recommended if treatment needs to be started before the fetus has any chance of survival. Also, termination may be considered in the first trimester if chemotherapy cannot wait until the second trimester and the risk of causing birth defects is considered to be unacceptably high. Even if these conditions are not present, some women will choose to terminate a desired pregnancy in order to wait until after treatment and their survival is more assured before starting or enlarging her family. And termination may be chosen by some women if the chances of survival are not good and the mother likely will not be around to see the child grow into adulthood, or there is no other adult in the family available who is capable of raising the child. Others may choose not to terminate even if carrying the pregnancy up to the time when the fetus can survive compromises their chances of survival. These are weighty concerns, which can cause a great deal of stress and worry about one's own mortality. But the patient can be directed to mental health and other support professionals to assist with decision-making and the stress involved.

MANAGEMENT OF THE PREGNANCY DURING CANCER TREATMENT

There are few changes to pregnancy management for a patient undergoing cancer treatment. If the condition is initially treated by surgery alone, pregnancy care is unchanged and any further treatment planned may be initiated after delivery. In this situation, delivery may be planned before 39 weeks' gestation so that the additional treatment can commence without further delay. If a patient is receiving chemotherapy, which significantly weakens the patient or causes a significant drop in blood counts, delivery can be timed for just before the next treatment is due in order to give the patient a chance to recover from her last treatment and for blood counts to return to normal. With either chemotherapy or radiation, ultrasound should be used to assess the fetus for growth restriction, and the patient may expect to receive more frequent ultrasounds to keep track of fetal progress and growth.

PREGNANCY AFTER CANCER

What about the patient who has been treated for cancer in the past—can she have a pregnancy? In most instances, the answer is yes if she is in remission. It is probably best to be without evidence of disease for at least a year before conceiving, and the patient should always check with her oncologist for her thoughts. But pregnancy does not appear to increase the chances of recurrence of cancer, even for those tumors that grow more when estrogen or progesterone are present (hormone receptor positive). In fact, a number of studies found better overall survival after hormone receptor positive breast cancer in those women who had a pregnancy after diagnosis and treatment.[7] Fertility after cancer treatment may be impaired, as chemotherapy and radiation treatments can cause the ovaries to stop releasing eggs. The heart and lungs can also have damage from some forms of chemotherapy, so these organs should be assessed prior to pregnancy. For the patient who is left infertile after treatment, IVF with a donor egg can be an option. Although there may be some changes to the size of the uterus and its inner lining from cancer treatment, the outcomes for pregnancy are similar to those women having IVF with a donor egg in terms of rates of pregnancy, miscarriage, and delivery of a living fetus.[8] Whether the conception occurs spontaneously or through IVF, management of the pregnancy without residual medical complications should not be different from that given to women without a history of cancer.

CASE STUDY #1

JoEllen was at 26 weeks' gestation when she noted a lump in her left breast. Her obstetrician referred her to a surgeon, who performed a biopsy, which showed cancer. She underwent both CT and MRI scans, which showed no evidence of spread outside the breast. After extensive counseling regarding prognosis and treatment during pregnancy, a recommendation was made to perform a lumpectomy with removal of a small number of lymph nodes to assess whether there was local spread of the tumor. These were performed and showed no evidence of tumor spread. A plan of care was made to give a round of chemotherapy every three weeks for the remainder of the pregnancy, when further assessment would be performed. During treatment she experienced hair loss and nausea for a few days after each round, but no other complications. Ultrasound studies showed that the fetus appeared to be growing at the 40th percentile, which was reasonable at this stage of the pregnancy and indicated continued growth. JoEllen received her last dose of chemotherapy at 35 weeks, and scheduled for labor induction three weeks later. The induction went without complication, and a healthy female infant was delivered with no signs of ill effects from the treatments. One week after delivery, JoEllen returned to her oncologist for a discussion regarding further assessment and treatment.

CASE STUDY #2

Josefina was at 22 weeks of gestation in her third pregnancy when she complained to her obstetrician that she was feeling unusually tired and was having a lot of bruising without trauma. A complete blood count (CBC) was performed, which showed anemia, a low platelet count, and a high percentage of immature white blood cells. She was referred to an oncologist, who recommended a bone marrow biopsy, which confirmed a diagnosis of acute myeloid leukemia (AML). Josefina was counseled that this is an aggressive cancer which would likely be fatal if not treated right away, and chemotherapy was recommended to start in the next week. She was then referred to a maternal-fetal medicine specialist for a discussion of the use of chemotherapy during pregnancy. At 24 weeks Josefina started a combination of chemotherapy drugs thought to be more appropriate for pregnancy, and she was noted to have a good response within the next six weeks as evidenced by improvement in her CBC. Fetal growth was monitored by ultrasound and continued to show normal. Fetal surveillance was initiated with non-stress tests (NSTs) at 32 weeks and were reassuring. However, at 34 weeks, it was noted that the CBC results were getting worse, and a discussion between the oncologist and the MFM resulted in a decision to deliver the pregnancy to allow for the initiation of additional medications with significant fetal risks. An induction of labor was performed, and a preterm female infant was delivered vaginally. The baby had some issues with jaundice, which resolved with two days of treatment with ultraviolet light, and was discharged from the neonatal ICU at three weeks of age. One week after delivery, Josefina was restarted on chemotherapy.

SUMMARY

A new diagnosis of cancer in a woman who is pregnant presents several challenges. The most important priority for the woman and the health care team is maximizing the chances of survival of the mother. Treatment may need to be started before the end of the pregnancy, and should not be postponed for concerns of fetal effects if it will compromise the woman's prognosis. Most chemotherapy agents given in the second and third trimester of pregnancy do not cause birth defects and are well tolerated by the fetus. Fetal growth should be monitored if chemotherapy is administered, and the baby should be evaluated after delivery for any ill effects, including anemia and suppression of the immune system. Yet most women receiving treatment for cancer during pregnancy will give birth to normal, healthy infants. The mother's prognosis will be dependent upon the type and stage of the cancer, and whether there is evidence of spread beyond the primary tumor, but should not be affected by the pregnancy.

PART IV

FETAL CONDITIONS

CHAPTER 15

BIRTH DEFECTS

MOST PEOPLE ARE SURPRISED to learn how common it is for a fetus to have a birth defect. Approximately 1 in every 33 babies (3%) is born with a birth defect, also referred to as a congenital fetal anomaly.[1] These anomalies can be in any organ system and most are very uncommon—less than 1 per 1,000 births. But when you add them all together, the chances of having at least one abnormality in some organ are not small. Most are sporadic and without an identifiable cause, while others can be related to genetic causes, medications, or underlying maternal diseases. They can be isolated, or with multiple present as part of a genetic syndrome. Birth defects can be of little clinical consequence, such as an extra rib or finger, routinely correctable with surgery, such as an intestinal blockage or cleft lip and palate (hole in the lip and roof of the mouth), surgically correctable and survivable in most situations, such as a diaphragmatic hernia (a hole in the diaphragm) or spina bifida (hole in the back where the spinal cord is exposed), or lethal, such as anencephaly (missing skull and brain) or absent kidneys. Some of the organ systems that can be affected are listed in box 15.1 with examples of abnormalities. Most structural birth defects are now detectable by ultrasound in the mid-second trimester.

BOX 15.1 EXAMPLES OF BIRTH DEFECTS IN DIFFERENT ORGAN SYSTEMS

- Nervous system
  - Absence of the skull and brain cortex (anencephaly)
  - Abnormal brain formation
  - Spina bifida (opening in the spine with the spinal cord exposed)
- Cardiac
  - Abnormal heart valve
  - Hole in the heart wall (septal defect)
  - Abnormal vessel connections
- Lungs
  - Cysts or growths in the lung tissue
  - Diaphragmatic hernia—a hole in the diaphragm allowing the intestines to enter the chest and push the lungs and heart to the side
  - Connections between the lungs and the esophagus (trachea-esophageal fistula)
- Face—cleft lip and palate (hole in the lip and roof of the mouth)
- Intestines—blockage (stenosis or atresia)
- Urinary system
  - Absence of one or both kidneys
  - Abnormal kidney tissue or cysts
  - Bladder outlet obstruction
- Skeletal
  - Fragile bones (osteogenesis imperfecta)
  - Extra or missing bones

- Dwarfism (achondroplasia)
- Deformities of the ankles (club feet)
- Neck
  - Fluid filled space behind the neck (cystic hygroma)
  - Other cysts in the front of the neck
- Genitals
  - Absent or malformed uterus
  - Undescended testes
  - Ambiguous genitalia
  - Urinary open on the side of the penis (hypospadias)
- Tumors
  - Teratoma
  - Neuroblastoma
  - Hemangioma

RISK FACTORS FOR AND TYPES OF BIRTH DEFECTS

The first risk factor for birth defects to discuss is having a close family history of an inheritable birth defect. These family-linked disorders are often referred to as multifactorial, meaning there is some component of both genetics and environment which contribute to the risk. And the risk is only elevated if the defect was present at birth for the mother, the father, or the sibling of the fetus. The risk is not elevated if the relative is more distant than either parent or a prior child. Defects in this category include neural tube defects such as spina bifida, heart defects, cleft lip and palate, and club foot. If there is a multifactorial defect in either parent or a sibling, the chances that the fetus will have the defect is 3–5%.[2]

There are certain genetic syndromes that can result in multiple anomalies being present. Having an extra chromosome 13 or 18 will result in the fetus having multiple anomalies, including but not limited to heart and brain abnormalities, cleft palate, and club feet. These syndromes often lead to miscarriage, premature birth, stillbirth, or death within the first year of life. Babies with DiGeorge syndrome (caused by missing part of chromosome 22) can have heart defects, kidney abnormalities, cleft lip and palate, hearing loss, and scoliosis, and they often develop psychiatric conditions such as anxiety and/or depression, autism spectrum disorder, and developmental delay. VACTERL is an acronym for another syndrome with many abnormalities, affecting some or all of the following: vertebrae, anus, heart (cardiac), trachea, esophagus, kidneys (renal), and limbs. Fortunately, the symptoms associated with VACTERL are usually not life threatening. Some of the defects do not impair function, while others may need surgical correction. Although some people born with VACTERL are more prone to chronic health issues, most go on to lead normal lives. The specific genetic abnormality for many but not all syndromes with multiple anomalies has now been identified, allowing for the diagnosis to be confirmed with a genetic test, either during fetal life (amniocentesis or CVS) or after birth. Syndromes such as these are very uncommon and not usually inherited from a parent, but rather they result from a problem with DNA replication during the fertilization process. As such, the risk of having a second child with the same syndrome is very low.

Birth defects can also be a result of a single gene defect inherited from one or both parents. Dominant disorders occur when a single abnormal gene is inherited from one parent with the condition, or the abnormal gene can arise without one of the parents being affected. This abnormal gene *dominates* over the gene on the other chromosome, causing the disorder, so there is no carrier state. Examples of dominant disorders causing birth defects are achondroplasia, where the primary feature is dwarfism, adult onset polycystic kidney disease, and polydactyly, where there is an extra finger on each hand. In contrast, recessive disorders occur when *both* parents are unaffected carriers, and the fetus inherits the abnormal gene from each parent. A recessive disorder that results in birth defects is childhood polycystic kidney disease, where normal kidney tissue in the fetus is replaced by nonfunctioning cysts. These genetic disorders will be discussed further in chapter 16.

Exposure of the fetus to certain conditions can also lead to birth defects. Maternal diabetes increases the risk of heart defects in the fetus, especially if the glucose control is poor in the first few weeks of pregnancy. Viral infections such as cytomegalovirus (CMV, discussed further in chapter 19) and rubella in the early part of pregnancy can cause multiple defects, such as blindness, deafness, heart defects, brain damage, and liver injury. Some seizure medications taken during pregnancy also increase the chances of having a baby with a birth defect. In particular, valproic acid (Depakote) increases the chances of spina bifida tenfold, and other seizure medications have been associated with increases in heart defects, facial changes, and fetal growth restriction.[3] Nonetheless, some seizure medication may still be needed, as seizures can be harmful to both the mother and the fetus. If possible, seizures should be controlled with a single medication which has a low risk of causing birth defects. Isotretinoin (Accutane), a medication taken for acne, causes birth defects in 35% or more of infants who are exposed during pregnancy, including small or absent ears, hearing and vision problems, heart defects, cleft palate, and fluid around the brain.[4] For this reason, isotretinoin is contraindicated for pregnancy and many controls are put in place to prevent its use by women who could become pregnant. Female users are required to take pregnancy tests every month during use of the drug, and must indicate the kind of birth control they are using if they are sexually active. If you are currently using a medication that has been associated with causing birth defects, be sure to discuss this with your health care practitioner prior to trying to conceive.

DIAGNOSIS OF BIRTH DEFECTS

The main way to diagnose birth defects during the pregnancy is ultrasound. Although some abnormalities can be evident earlier in the pregnancy, the best time to use ultrasound to look for birth defects is between 18 and 22 weeks. This is the time when the organs are large enough to be able to distinguish between normal and abnormal structures. However, not all anomalies are evident on ultrasound at this point in the pregnancy, and some anomalies cannot be identified by ultrasound at any time. A normal mid-trimester should be very reassuring but is not a guarantee that an anomaly will not be recognized later.

MANAGEMENT OF BIRTH DEFECTS

When a birth defect is identified by ultrasound, the next step should be to arrange appropriate counseling. Depending upon the defect and resources available, this counseling can be performed by a geneticist, a maternal-fetal medicine specialist, a pediatric specialist, or a combination of these specialists. Pediatric specialists might include cardiologists, surgeons, and neonatologists. The counseling should consist of a description of what has been identified, possible causes, implications for management of the rest of the pregnancy and delivery, and the prognosis for the child both short and long term. Counseling might suggest other tests which could elucidate the cause and extent of the problem, and whether there are any treatments available during the pregnancy that can improve the outcome. It may be that the delivery should occur at a hospital with highly skilled specialists to give the baby the best chance of survival. Counseling may also include a discussion of the options of pregnancy termination versus carrying the pregnancy to term. If surgical correction after delivery is possible, the procedure with its risks and benefits should be described, as well as what the recovery period will entail. The patient should also be informed as to whether the defect is sporadic, or whether future pregnancies are at increased risk for a recurrence. This counseling can be quite complex, and having a case manager sometimes referred to as a patient navigator can often be helpful in answering questions and making the necessary decisions and arrangements.

INTRAUTERINE SURGERY FOR BIRTH DEFECTS

We have now entered an era where correction of some birth defects is possible with the baby still inside the uterus. *In utero* surgery allows for correction of a problem before the fetus deteriorates further while allowing the pregnancy to continue and lessen the risks of prematurity. The most commonly performed in utero surgery now for a fetal anomaly is spina bifida repair. Not all babies with spina bifida are candidates for this procedure, and it is only available in bigger cities with major medical centers. The procedure is only performed between 19 and 26 weeks, and if the opening is in the lower portion of the fetal spine. Under general anesthesia for the mother, an incision is made in her abdomen over the uterus, and an operating scope is inserted into the uterus near the defect. Sutures are then placed in the skin on both sides of the opening and the sides are pulled together closing the defect. Studies have shown that this procedure can result in better function of the bowels, bladder, and legs than closing the defect after the baby is born, and it reduces the chances of needing a tube placed in the brain (shunt) to drain excess fluid.[5] There are risks to this procedure, however; if an incision is placed in the uterus to perform the repair rather than using a scope, the mother will need a cesarean for this and all future pregnancies, and the uterine scar could rupture in future pregnancies. For the fetus, the main risk is that the procedure could lead to infection and increases the chances of preterm birth, and the baby may still be left with disabilities. Thorough counseling regarding the risks and benefits of the procedure is important for the parents to make an informed choice. Some decide that they do not want the procedure and opt for termination or waiting until after delivery for surgical repair.

There are other in utero procedures being attempted to improve the outcomes for fetal anomalies. One is for diaphragmatic hernia, where a scope is placed through the mother's abdomen and into the uterus to insert a balloon into the fetal trachea (windpipe) to reduce pressure on the fetal lungs and allow for better lung development. When there is a blockage in the bladder outlet, a catheter can be inserted into the fetal bladder to reduce overextension, preserving bladder and kidney function. A shunt can be placed into the fetal chest if an abnormal fluid collection is compressing one or both lungs. These procedures are more experimental in nature in that the benefits are not clear and are only available in a few centers around the country.

CASE STUDY #1

Margarita was referred to a maternal-fetal medicine specialist after an ultrasound at 20 weeks revealed that the fetus had spina bifida. A detailed ultrasound was performed confirming an opening in the lower spine with evidence of excess fluid around the brain often seen with this type of spinal defect. No other abnormalities were detected. Prior genetic testing had shown a very low risk of a chromosome defect. The types of disabilities associated with spina bifida were discussed with Margarita and her partner, which included the possibility of incontinence and being unable to walk. They were then referred for further counseling with a pediatric neurosurgeon, who discussed the options of closing the spinal defect after delivery versus during the pregnancy. After consideration of the risks and benefits of both approaches, Margarita consented to the operation with the baby still in the uterus. At 22 weeks, Margarita underwent general anesthesia, and an incision was made in her abdomen to expose her upper uterus. An operating scope was then inserted into the uterus and the spinal defect was visualized. Instruments were then inserted through the scope to sew the defect closed so that the spinal cord was no longer exposed to the amniotic fluid. After a short stay in the hospital postoperatively she was discharged, and follow-up ultrasounds showed resolution of the excess fluid around the brain. At 37 weeks she went into spontaneous labor and delivered a 7-pound female infant vaginally without complication. At the age of 3, the child was walking normally and was continent.

CASE STUDY #2

Jolee was at 20 weeks' gestation when an ultrasound showed the fetus had a diaphragmatic hernia. A section of the small bowel protruded through the hole in the diaphragm into the chest, pushing the heart to the right side of the chest and compressing the lungs. No other fetal anomalies were noted. She was first referred to a pediatric cardiologist for a cardiac echo because of the increased risk of associated heart defects, and then referred to a pediatric surgeon for counseling about the condition and its implications. Specifically, the fetus would need surgery soon after delivery to return the bowel to the abdomen and close the diaphragm defect. A survival rate of 60–70% was given, and would depend on whether the lungs had enough room to grow and develop before birth. She also met with a physician from the neonatal intensive care unit (NICU) to discuss what the care would be like after surgery.

Frequent ultrasounds were performed for the rest of the pregnancy to check for complications, but none developed. At 39 weeks

Jolee had a cesarean delivery because the fetus was breech, and the infant was taken immediately to the NICU for stabilization. Soon after, the baby girl was taken to the operating room, where the defect was repaired, and then returned to the NICU. She stayed on a ventilator for four weeks and was eventually discharged with a home oxygen requirement, which she eventually outgrew and no longer needed. Jolee was counseled that the chance that a diaphragmatic hernia would recur in a future pregnancy was 1–2%.

SUMMARY

Congenital fetal anomalies are not rare, and they can affect almost any organ in the developing fetus. Identification is most often made by ultrasound in the mid-second trimester, and a determination needs to be made as to whether the defect is isolated or part of a syndrome. Counseling should then be given to the patient regarding the extent of the problem, possible causes, implications for the remainder of the pregnancy, the prognosis, and management options. With this information, the patient will be better prepared to make decisions about her pregnancy, about treatment options available for the fetus or newborn, and about lifestyle changes and care that may be necessary when the baby is born. Every situation is different, of course, and the needs of families and access to adequate care can impact the choices available and the decisions women and their partners make when a diagnosis is offered.

CHAPTER 16

GENETIC ABNORMALITIES

IN THE PREVIOUS CHAPTER, one type of genetic abnormality was discussed, namely, those that are associated with structural abnormalities of the fetus. In this chapter, genetic abnormalities that affect all cells in the body of the fetus will be discussed. This will include whole chromosomal abnormalities as well as single-gene abnormalities, some of which also cause structural abnormalities.

The DNA of humans consists of 23 pairs of chromosomes, with one of each pair inherited from each parent. The joining of the chromosomes from the parents which will comprise the DNA makeup of the fetus occurs at the time of conception. Each chromosome contains hundreds to thousands of genes, which code for all of the traits that the child will exhibit. Each gene is made up of a sequence of base pairs, often numbering in the thousands. For each gene there is a standard sequence of these base pairs, but on occasion there is a change in one or more of the base pairs. When this change causes a problem in the function of the gene, it is called a mutation. When it does not change the function of the gene, it is called a variant, and is of little or no significance. For most genes, the standard sequence is dominant, meaning that it will perform as expected even if the gene inherited from the other parent is a variant or a mutation. In this case, the variant or mutation will be recessive, and unexpressed. Using sickle cell as an example, if a normal hemoglobin gene is inherited from one parent but a sickle gene from the other parent, the child will not have sickle cell disease, since the normal hemoglobin gene is dominant. Instead, the child will be a carrier of the disorder but unaffected. The child would only have the disorder if he inherited the abnormal recessive gene from both parents who are carriers. It should be noted that some recessive disorders can be lethal in the neonatal or early childhood periods, such as Tay-Sachs and Gaucher disease, making prenatal genetic testing valuable for many couples.

WHOLE CHROMOSOME ABNORMALITIES

As mentioned above, during the fertilization process at the time of conception, the fetus will get one of the pair from each parent for each of the 23 chromosomes, thought to be on a random basis. However, on occasion, there will be an error in this process, and the fetus can receive an extra chromosome from either the father or the mother. This is referred to as trisomy. The trisomy that people are most familiar with is having an extra chromosome 21, or trisomy 21, also known as Down syndrome. Half of babies with Down syndrome have major birth defects of the heart, and all have some degree of mental disability as well as other health issues. Down syndrome is actually the mildest form of trisomy. Fetuses with trisomy 13 or 18 all have multiple severe major anomalies that can include club feet, holes in the heart, cysts in the brain, or the growth of some organs outside the body. Trisomy 13 and 18 are usually incompatible with survival, meaning that there is a high rate of miscarriage or stillbirth, and less than 10% of babies born alive with trisomy 13 or 18 survive to their first birthday. With trisomy of other chromosomes, the result is usually loss of the pregnancy in the first trimester. Other chromosomal abnormalities include having an extra part of a chromosome, or missing a part of a chromosome. Examples include DiGeorge syndrome (discussed in chapter 15), associated with congenital heart disease, impairment of the immune system, and developmental delay. Prader-Willi syndrome results from a deletion of part of chromosome 15 but does not cause birth defects. It is associated with feeding difficulties in infancy, weak muscles with low tone, short stature, developmental delay, and difficulty controlling emotions. Having an extra copy of part of chromosome 7 can lead to heart problems, delayed development, and weak muscle tone. The clinical picture of structural defects, mental development, and long-term survival will be determined by which chromosome is affected, and how much of that chromosome is missing or extra.

SINGLE-GENE ABNORMALITIES

Also discussed briefly in chapter 15, mutations of a single gene can result in a birth defect, but they can also be associated with a disease without a defect. Cystic fibrosis and sickle cell anemia are examples of disorders caused by defects in a single gene where no structural anomalies are present at birth. A recessive disorder is when the condition requires two abnormal genes to be inherited, one from each parent. In this situation, both parents would be carriers and not affected if they have a second normal gene. A dominant disorder is when a person is affected with only one abnormal gene, either inherited from an affected parent, or from a new mutation which is not inherited. Cystic fibrosis and sickle cell anemia are both recessive disorders, while dwarfism (achondroplasia) and adult polycystic kidney disease are examples of dominant disorders.

REPEAT EXPANSION DISORDERS

There are situations where a sequence in the DNA repeats itself when there is only supposed to be one copy. If a limited number of repeats is present, this situation is usually asymptomatic. Over generations, however, the number of times the sequence is repeated can grow and cause gene disruptions with resulting disease. Most often these diseases are neurologic in nature and often are not clinically apparent at birth. Huntington's disease is caused by excessive repeats on chromosome 4, and symptoms can include uncontrollable movement, mental health changes, and cognitive decline usually beginning in the fourth and fifth decades of life. Fragile X is due to an excess in repeats on the X chromosome and can result in intellectual disability, behavior and learning challenges, and unusual features including a narrow face, large ears, and a prominent forehead.

TESTING FOR GENETIC DISORDERS

Testing for both whole-chromosome and single-gene genetic disorders was discussed in chapter 4. Genetic screening should be offered to all patients, and is usually discussed at the first prenatal visit. As previously mentioned, testing for whole-chromosome abnormalities can be performed through serum screening, cell-free DNA testing, or direct testing with CVS or amniocentesis. Serum screening and cell-free DNA testing are considered *screening* tests, since they only detect increased probability of having an abnormality and require further testing for confirmation, while both CVS and amniocentesis are considered *diagnostic* tests, as they give a definitive answer as to whether an abnormality is present. If you receive a positive screening, usually the next step is a diagnostic one, if you choose to have further testing.

For single-gene abnormalities, a blood test can be performed which determines whether a person is a carrier and can pass an abnormal gene to the fetus. Different companies offer tests that screen for hundreds of these gene disorders. If the mother is screened and is found to be a carrier for one or more of these conditions, testing should then be offered to the partner to determine if he is also a carrier for the same disorder. If both parents are carriers, there is a 50% chance that one parent will pass the abnormal gene on to the fetus, and a 25% chance that the fetus will inherit the abnormal gene from both parents and be affected by the condition. To determine whether a fetus is a carrier for or affected by the condition where both parents are carriers, cells will then need to be collected from the fetus, either by CVS or amniocentesis, to determine whether the fetus has inherited none, one, or both abnormal genes from the parents.

Testing for repeat expansion disorders is now also possible. If a parent has Huntington's disease, each child has a 50% chance of developing this disorder; if testing shows more than 40 copies of the abnormal sequence, they will develop the disorder. Fragile X syndrome can only be inherited from the mother, and 50% of male children will be affected. During the prenatal period the mother can be tested for the number of repeats of the sequence that causes Fragile X. If she has more than 55 copies but less than 200 repeats, she has the premutation, and her children are at risk. Those with a premutation should be offered CVS or amniocentesis, where fetal DNA will be obtained and tested to see if more than 200 repeats are present and the fetus will be affected.

MANAGEMENT OF ABNORMAL GENETIC TEST RESULTS

If a genetic abnormality has been detected in the fetus, counseling with an expert in the disorder is usually the next step. During this counseling the nature of the disorder is discussed along with its prognosis and possible treatments. What is usually recognized is that there is a spectrum of manifestations for most disorders, so the exact clinical course may be difficult to predict. Every fetus is different, and every expectant mother is different. The genetic counseling is complex; asking questions at this counseling is expected and taking notes is advised. A good counselor will listen carefully to your concerns and respond patiently to your questions. Implications for future pregnancies should also be discussed. With this information, the parents can be better prepared to make decisions. Some parents may choose to pursue pregnancy termination for serious disorders, while others can choose to continue the pregnancy with the knowledge of how the child's care can be managed after delivery. In the wake of the overturning of the *Roe v. Wade* decision in 2022, which protected a woman's right to choose abortion, laws can vary from state to state, so it's important to discuss what options might be available to you in your state.

The whole-chromosomal disorders described above occur by random chance. They are neither preventable nor caused by anything the mother or father did. Because they are random, the good news is that they are highly unlikely to occur again. In addition, the future holds the possibility that some gene disorders can be treated before birth with stem cell transplants or other interventions that can alter the course of the condition, but this is not currently an option.

If it is recognized before pregnancy that both parents are a carrier for a recessive single-gene defect, IVF may be an option. Even if the couple is not infertile, IVF would give them the option of creating multiple embryos and testing each one for the gene defect. Embryos found to be free of the disorder can then be identified and only they are used for implantation into the uterus, eliminating the chances of having an affected child.

Sometimes, a genetic diagnosis can impact the health of the mother, making delivery more challenging or introducing new impacts on health concerns the mother may already have. Carrying a baby that is destined to die shortly after birth can have mental health implications even for those who have not suffered with mental health challenges before. The challenge of raising a disabled child can also present mental, physical, and financial challenges parents may wish to consider during this time.

CASE STUDY #1

At her first prenatal visit, Joannie was offered genetic testing and she opted for cell-free DNA testing and carrier screening. The cell-free test reduced her chances of the fetus having a whole-chromosome defect from 1 in 200 based on her age to 1 in 3,000, but the carrier screen showed that she was a carrier for Tay-Sachs disease, a severe neurologic condition where the child progressively deteriorates and often dies by the age of 5. Her partner, Paul, was then tested and also found to be a carrier for Tay-Sachs. This meant that the fetus had a 50% chance of also being a carrier, but also a 25% chance of being affected. The couple decided to have CVS testing, and the DNA testing of the cells obtained by CVS showed that the fetus had two abnormal genes at the Tay-Sachs location. This meant that the child would be affected by the disease. Joannie and Paul were counseled by a geneticist regarding the likelihood of the child being severely affected and dying at an early age, and they decided to terminate the pregnancy. To prevent this from happening again, six months later they pursued IVF with preimplantation genetic testing to eliminate the risk of having another affected child. Twelve embryos were obtained through IVF, and testing revealed that three had both abnormal genes, four had one abnormal gene and would be carriers, and five had no genes for Tay-Sachs. One of the normal embryos was transferred successfully, and Joannie went on to have a normal pregnancy and a healthy baby. She did this two more times, and now has three healthy children.

CASE STUDY #2

Seema was born with phenylketonuria (PKU), an inherited disorder caused by the inability to break down the amino acid phenylalanine, which is present in all food containing protein. Levels of phenylalanine then rise in the bloodstream, which can lead to intellectual and developmental disabilities if not recognized during infancy. Seema was identified as having PKU by screening performed at all hospitals in the United States, and begun on a diet with very little protein. She followed this diet well at first, but during her teen years she was not as compliant. She was counseled that, were she to get pregnant, it would be very important for her to be back on the strict diet and have near normal blood levels of phenylalanine in early pregnancy to protect the fetus even if it did not have the disease itself.

Seema became strictly compliant with the low-protein diet when she was planning pregnancy, and conceived after her phenylalanine level was in an acceptable range. Her partner was tested and did not carry the gene for PKU, so it was concluded that the fetus would be a carrier (Seema only had abnormal genes to pass to the fetus) for PKU but not affected by the disorder. Seema continued to follow the diet as best she could during the entire pregnancy, and frequent phenylalanine level testing remained reassuring. She went on to deliver a healthy male infant, and subsequent testing confirmed that the boy did not have PKU. As of age 2, he was meeting all developmental milestones.

SUMMARY

Independent of maternal age, all women are at some risk of having a child with a genetic abnormality. With genetic testing, it is possible to know whether this risk is elevated or quite low. If the mother is identified as a carrier for a serious disorder, further testing is available to determine whether the fetus will be affected. For whole-chromosome abnormalities, screening tests are also available to determine the level of risk, but such abnormalities, if found to be present, can be very serious and can have negative outcomes. Patients should decide whether they are interested in testing, and if so which test is right for them. If an abnormality in the fetus is identified, counseling is available to discuss the meaning of the abnormality and the range of possible clinical manifestations, treatment options, and delivery options.

CHAPTER 17

FETAL CARDIAC ARRHYTHMIAS

THE FETAL HEART forms early in pregnancy, with a heartbeat routinely detectable with ultrasound four weeks after conception. As the pregnancy progresses, the heart rate becomes more stable between 120 and 160 beats per minute, usually toward the slower part of this range in the third trimester. With the small size of the heart, it needs a rate this high to deliver oxygen and other nutrients to the tissue in sufficient amounts for the fetus to thrive.

Later in pregnancy, however, abnormalities in the rhythm of the fetal heartbeat can, on occasion, be detected. The rate can be overly fast, slow, or irregular. Many of these abnormalities are tolerated by the fetus and some resolve spontaneously after delivery. An irregular rhythm is the best example of this, especially if due to premature atrial contractions. But some abnormal rhythms interfere with the heart's ability to function properly. An overly fast heart rate (tachycardia) may not give the heart enough time between beats to refill with blood before the next heartbeat, so the cardiac output drops. Fetal hyperthyroidism or anemia, infection, maternal fever, and some drugs can cause this issue, but often it is a condition inherent to the heart itself called supraventricular tachycardia (SVT). An overly slow heart rate (bradycardia) can also result in a drop in cardiac output with insufficient oxygen delivery to the rest of the body. Fetal bradycardia can be a result of an immune disorder, a heart defect, or an abnormality in the electrical connections in the heart.

IRREGULAR FETAL HEART RATES

When listening to the fetal heart rate, on occasion an irregular rhythm will be heard. It can be an early beat followed by a pause, or a skipped beat. This should generate an ultrasound examination of the heart to make sure it is structurally normal. If no heart defects are discovered and the heart muscle appears to be functioning well, this irregular rhythm is almost always benign, and frequently the irregularity resolves after delivery. No further investigation is needed and the rest of the pregnancy care can be routine.

FETAL TACHYCARDIA

Fetal tachycardia is more concerning than an irregular rhythm. When a fetal heart rate greater than 180 is detected in the absence of obvious maternal infection or fever, further investigation is warranted. First, it is important to use ultrasound to perform a Doppler study of an artery in the brain to determine whether the rapid heart rate is due to fetal anemia. If this Doppler study is normal, the rhythm of the heart is evaluated to determine where in the heart the tachycardia is originating. The most common cause of fetal tachycardia is SVT, where the abnormal rhythm originates in the atrium, and the atrium and ventricle are beating at the same fast rate. With SVT, it is then important to determine how much of the time the heart is in the high range, as it can switch back and forth between a normal rate and a high rate. The more time the heart is in SVT, the more it will interfere with the heart's ability to supply oxygen and other nutrients to the rest of the body. If the heart stays in SVT 100% of the time, the situation can then evolve into fetal hydrops, where the fetus retains fluid due to heart failure. This will be discussed more in chapter 20.

When SVT is persistent, and signs develop that show the heart is beginning to fail, medication is given to the mother which will cross into the fetal circulation. Most often, digoxin is the first medication tried, but it requires careful monitoring to make sure the mother does not develop complications. The administration of this medication is frequently done on an inpatient basis, as the digoxin dose needs to be increased slowly. Digoxin levels need to be monitored frequently, and the mother's cardiac rhythm needs to be assessed for signs of toxicity. Once a therapeutic level of digoxin is reached, an evaluation will determine if the SVT has converted to normal sinus rhythm; if not, a second medication may be added. Often, this second medication will be effective in getting the rhythm to convert, but close monitoring of the mother and fetus are still necessary, and both medications may need to be continued for the remainder of the pregnancy. On occasion, the medication does not cross the placenta well, and it will need to be given through a needle directly into the fetus under ultrasound guidance. If medications are not able to return the fetus to normal sinus rhythm, and heart function is deteriorating, delivery may be necessary to prevent stillbirth, and the same medications may be more effective given directly to the fetus in the neonatal ICU. Without control of the tachycardia, heart failure will likely ensue, and potentially fetal death.

FETAL BRADYCARDIA

A very slow fetal heart rate can be caused either by a heart defect or by autoimmune antibodies in the mother that cross into the fetal circulation. These antibodies are found in most patients with Sjogren's syndrome (an autoimmune disorder causing dry eyes and mouth and sometimes affecting the kidneys) and some patients with systemic lupus or other autoimmune disorders (discussed in chapter 9). The particular antibodies are named anti-SS-A and anti-SS-B, and they can cross the placenta into the fetal circulation starting in the early second trimester. Therefore, pregnant women with autoimmune disorders should be screened during pregnancy for the presence of these antibodies, and if one or both antibodies are detected the patient should be monitored for the development of bradycardia. In less than 5% of patients with these antibodies, they attach to cells in the heart that control the baby's heart rate and cause the rate to slow. However, this slowing occurs in as many as 20% of women who have had a previous fetus with antibody-mediated bradycardia. The fetus may tolerate this slow rate and still be able to supply sufficient oxygen and nutrients to the body, but the situation must be monitored closely for the remainder of the pregnancy to ensure that the slow rate does not lead to a deterioration in cardiac function. If this deterioration were to occur, the damage to the heart may be permanent, and premature delivery may become necessary to avoid fetal death. During labor, the slow heart rate will not allow interpretation of the heart rate pattern on the monitor; in this situation a cesarean delivery is usually performed rather than having the labor unmonitored. After delivery, this slow rate will likely lead to the need for the baby to have a pacemaker, as bradycardia will not allow for the delivery of sufficient blood flow and nutrients as the baby grows and becomes more active.

Some patients with no known autoimmune disease will be found to have a fetus with bradycardia. Tests for anti-SS-A and anti-SS-B should be performed as well as a fetal echocardiogram to determine the cause. About 50% of patients with fetal bradycardia but no known autoimmune disorder will be found to have one or both of these antibodies, and many of these women will develop an autoimmune disorder within the next few years. These pregnancies should be managed similarly to pregnancies of women with known autoimmune disorders and fetal bradycardia.

Some physicians advocate screening all patients with the anti-SS-A and anti-SS-B antibodies with fetal echocardiogram every week between 16 and 26 weeks of pregnancy. The idea is to catch signs that the fetal heart is showing abnormalities before full bradycardia develops, and to treat them with high-dose steroids to prevent progression. However, bradycardia will only develop in less than 5% of pregnancies with these antibodies, fetal echocardiograms are expensive and not always available, the steroids cause blood sugar levels to rise, and the data that bradycardia can be prevented or reversed are not strong. Alternatively, the pregnancy can be followed by documenting the fetal heart rate in the office every two weeks, with referral to a pediatric cardiologist if bradycardia does develop.

CASE STUDY #1

Rishi was at an appointment at 32 weeks in her first pregnancy when her physician heard a very rapid fetal heart rate. An ultrasound was performed which demonstrated a fetal heart rate of 240 and no cardiac anomalies. Rishi was admitted to the hospital and a pediatric cardiologist was consulted. As the rate remained around 240 for the first three hours, a decision was made to start Rishi on digoxin. She did not have any side effects, but it took two days to achieve an appropriate blood level. An echocardiogram was performed daily and continued to show good function of the fetal heart but the rate remained over 220 all of the time. A second medication was started, but the rate remained high, and after two days there were signs of developing hydrops. A course of antenatal steroids was started to advance fetal lung maturation should premature delivery be needed, and a needle was inserted into the fetal buttocks under ultrasound guidance and the medication was injected into the muscle. After 48 hours, there was still no change in the tachycardia, and an echocardiogram now showed poor contractility of the heart muscle. A cesarean delivery was performed, and a 34-week female fetus weighing 5 pounds was delivered and taken to the neonatal ICU. The baby was given medications to slow the heart rate through an IV and did respond after two days with slowing of the heart rate to 160. Heart muscle contractility also improved and by day seven of life was thought to be normal. She experienced mild respiratory distress initially due to prematurity, and needed oxygen therapy for the first three days. On day 10 of life she was deemed stable on medication, and discharged with a repeat echocardiogram scheduled in one week.

CASE STUDY #2

At the age of 19, Luisa was diagnosed with Sjogren's syndrome after complaining to her primary care physician about dry eyes and a dry mouth. At the time, she was noted to have SS-A and SS-B antibodies in her blood, and hydroxychloroquine was prescribed. She conceived at the age of 27, at a time when her Sjogren's symptoms were still well controlled. When she went to her first prenatal visit, the presence of these antibodies was confirmed and continuation of hydroxychloroquine was recommended. She was told that she would be at risk for the fetus developing bradycardia due to these antibodies, and that monitoring the fetal heart rate more closely would be necessary. At 16 weeks, she was asked to have office visits every two weeks so that the fetal heart rate could be ascertained. At 22 weeks, the fetal heart rate was noted to have dropped to 80 from 130 at her prior visit, and an appointment was scheduled with a pediatric cardiologist the following week. At this appointment, the fetal heart rate was noted to be 72, with normal heart structure and good movement of the ventricles. Luisa had echocardiograms repeated every two weeks after that showing a stable heart rate in the 70s and good heart function. Monthly ultrasound measurements also showed that the fetus was growing normally.

The pregnancy continued to term without any new concerns, and a cesarean delivery was performed at 39 weeks given that the fetal heart rate was too low for monitoring during labor. The baby did well in the nursery, but ultimately needed placement of a pacemaker.

SUMMARY

When an abnormal fetal heart rate is detected, evaluation of the cause is needed to determine the best approach to therapy. With fetal tachycardia, causes including hyperthyroidism and fetal anemia need to be excluded. If SVT is present, intensive medication treatment given to the mother most often works to control the heart rate before deterioration of heart function occurs. With fetal bradycardia, blood work will determine if it is caused by autoimmune antibodies, and ultrasound can identify heart anomalies which could be the cause. Continued monitoring of the fetal heart function is performed for both fast- and slow-rate abnormalities. If heart function remains good, the prognosis for the pregnancy is also good.

CHAPTER 18

FETAL GROWTH RESTRICTION

THROUGH A COMBINATION of both nutrition and genetic programming, a fetus grows steadily throughout pregnancy, with the biggest weight gain occurring in the third trimester. The median birth weight at full term is about 7½ pounds, with male infants weighing slightly more than female infants on average. Birth weight is considered normal if it is between the 10th and 90th percentile for a population, which at term is roughly 5½ and 8½ pounds in the United States. Babies larger than this are termed macrosomic, or large for gestational age. Babies smaller than this are termed growth restricted, or small for gestational age. Sometimes the abbreviation *IUGR* is used, which stands for intrauterine growth restriction.

When macrosomia is present, there is an increased risk of cesarean, shoulder dystocia (where the head delivers but the shoulders and body are stuck in the birth canal), and maternal vaginal tears. The baby is at risk for birth injuries such as broken arms and nerve damage, low blood sugar in the newborn period, and developing obesity and type II diabetes later in life. Small for gestational age babies are at risk for health, growth, and developmental issues in childhood, including cognitive delay, hyperactivity, and cerebral palsy. And there is evidence now that fetal growth restriction increases the chances of a person developing hypertension, type II diabetes, and heart disease in adulthood. This chapter will focus on the diagnosis and management of growth delay, which starts during fetal life.

RISK FACTORS FOR FETAL GROWTH RESTRICTION

Risk factors for fetal growth restriction can be divided into three categories: maternal, fetal, and placental. Maternal risk factors include hypertension, preeclampsia, autoimmune disorders, previous pregnancy with growth restriction, smoking, low maternal weight, and some other chronic diseases. Fetal factors which can lead to fetal growth restriction include multiple gestation, chromosomal abnormalities, birth defects, congenital infections (see chapter 19), and some genetic syndromes. Placental factors include bleeding behind the placenta, chronic abruption, and when the umbilical cord is abnormally inserted into the placenta. Identifying a cause may be helpful for management decisions. Very few of these are modifiable, but growth restriction due to fetal or placental factors usually does not recur in future pregnancies.

ASSESSMENT OF FETAL GROWTH

Assessment of fetal growth is an important part of prenatal care. Some indication of fetal growth can be obtained by measuring the height of the uterus at prenatal visits, but a better assessment can be made by ultrasound. In the second half of pregnancy, measurements of the fetal head, femur, and abdominal circumference are routinely made during the ultrasound examination, and a formula is then used to generate the estimated fetal weight (EFW). Tables are then used to determine the EFW percentile for the particular gestational age when the scan is being performed. When the ultrasound EFW is less than the 10th percentile, the fetus is considered growth restricted. However, the calculation of the EFW is not precise. The EFW is within 20% of the actual weight 95% of the time; the other 5% of the time it is off by more than 20%.

In addition to the measurement of the above parameters, the ultrasound will also assess the amount of amniotic fluid surrounding the fetus, as well as the blood flow through an umbilical cord artery at the end of the heartbeat (diastolic flow) using the Doppler technique. Reduction in the amount of amniotic fluid, or elevation of the Doppler readings in the umbilical artery, are associated with increased risk of perinatal mortality.

The fetus can be below the population's overall 10th percentile without there being a problem. Some ethnic groups tend to have smaller babies, and smaller parents also tend to have smaller babies. In these instances the fetus may be achieving its appropriate genetic growth potential. In these situations the amniotic fluid level remains normal and the Doppler reading is in the normal range. But at least half the time, the fetus is small due to a problem. The fetus may not be getting the nutrients it needs, so it slows its growth to conserve energy for the function of vital organs, including the heart and brain. As a reflection of this, we often will see the abdominal circumference at a much lower percentile than the other measurement due to less growth in the abdominal organs. If this situation of reduced delivery of nutrients to the fetus continues to progress over a long period of time, it can lead to deterioration in the condition of the fetus, possibly leading to stillbirth if delivery does not occur.

MANAGEMENT OF FETAL GROWTH RESTRICTION

When an ultrasound demonstrates fetal growth restriction, management decisions will depend on the cause, the gestational age, and the condition of the fetus. Testing for genetic abnormalities, antiphospholipid antibodies, and congenital infections should be considered in an effort to identify the cause. If the growth restriction is due to inadequate nutrients passing from the mother to the fetus (i.e., not fetal factors), the ability of the fetus to compensate with slowing of growth may be exceeded and it may be at risk for deterioration. Increasing the mother's caloric intake will not correct the problem; nor will increasing her amount of bed rest. If the pregnancy is far enough along that the parents would want to intervene to prevent stillbirth (usually starting around 24 weeks if growth restriction is present), tests of fetal well-being are initiated. The first test done is either a non-stress test (NST) or a biophysical profile (BPP), usually on a weekly basis, along with umbilical artery assessment by Doppler. The NST and BPP were described in chapter 6. As long as these tests remain reassuring, the pregnancy is continued, feeling that the risks of prematurity outweigh the very low risk of stillbirth. But when the fetus reaches term, starting at 37 weeks, delivery is routinely recommended rather than letting the pregnancy progress past the due date.

This level of fetal surveillance is almost always sufficient to allow for delivery before fetal well-being is compromised. You should be reassured that there is a usual pattern of progression of findings as the fetus becomes sicker. The first step would be elevated Doppler readings of the umbilical artery. Second would come a nonreactive NST, followed by loss of fetal breathing movements as part of the BPP. Then there would be a decrease in the amount of amniotic fluid surrounding the fetus. This can be followed by absent or reverse diastolic flow in the umbilical artery by Doppler. Most likely then the mother would perceive a decrease in fetal movements. Fetal monitoring would then demonstrate decelerations or other abnormalities occurring in the fetal heart rate. The earlier the pregnancy is, the farther along this pathway your caregiver would allow this pregnancy to continue before committing to delivery. Closer to term, delivery would be recommended earlier in the progression. In general, delivery is recommended between 34 and 37 weeks with abnormal findings such as decreased amniotic fluid or absent diastolic flow in the umbilical artery, earlier if the flow is reversed. Not all fetuses will follow this order, but parents should be reassured the earlier you are in this pathway that stillbirth is very unlikely to occur. If concerning signs are present and delivery before 34 weeks is likely, antenatal corticosteroids are given to improve lung maturation and reduce the risk of prematurity complications.

How often should the ultrasound be repeated to determine if a fetus is getting further behind in growth? It depends on how far below the 10th percentile the growth is. In general, ultrasound measurements are repeated every 3–4 weeks, but no more frequently than 14 days, as the inherent variations in measurements will make assessment of growth less accurate. As stated previously, the NST or BPP are repeated weekly, but more frequently if other concerning factors are present.

If the growth restriction is due to inadequate delivery of nutrients to the fetus, it would be reasonable to think that the outcome for the baby would be better if it did not progress as far in signs of deterioration. That is, deliver the growth-retarded fetus before the Doppler study is abnormal. However, two studies looked at this question, both finding that earlier delivery did not improve outcome.[1]

Multiple gestation pregnancies are at specific risk for at least one fetus developing growth restriction, with 25–50% of fetuses being below the 10th percentile. It is twice as common in identical twins sharing a placenta relative to fraternal twins.[2] The uterus has the capability of nourishing twins normally until about 32 weeks, at which point we routinely see the growth curves of twins diverge from that of singletons. It can be thought of as the combined needs of the fetuses now being greater than what the uterus can supply. As such, most twins born near term have a birth weight between the 10th and 50th percentiles for singletons. If one or both fall below the 10th percentile, the pregnancy is managed similarly to a single pregnancy with a growth-restricted fetus. However, if the blood supply is not distributed equally to both twins, one can develop growth restriction earlier and fetal surveillance should be started. On occasion, a decision will need to be made to move to delivery because the smaller twin is showing signs of compromise, including the cessation of growth. In this situation, because it is not possible to deliver only the smaller one, the normally grown twin will be exposed to the risks of prematurity even though it was doing well inside the uterus.

Fetuses that are growth restricted have twice the odds of needing a cesarean delivery.[3] The growth-restricted fetus has less reserve for tolerating the stress of labor, especially with more severe restriction, and fetal deterioration can be manifested by abnormalities on the fetal heart rate tracing. But most fetuses with growth restriction do have enough reserve to tolerate labor and delivery vaginally. The mother's recovery should not be affected by growth restriction, and she is discharged at the normal time after delivery.

Once the growth-restricted fetus is delivered, it is evaluated by the pediatrics team. If needed, resuscitation measures will be instituted in the delivery room. The need for resuscitative measures will be greater with the degree of prematurity and the growth restriction. When the fetus is stable, it will be weighed. Since the diagnosis of growth restriction is based on estimates made by ultrasound and some degree of inaccuracy is therefore likely, the birth weight will then be checked on a chart to determine whether the weight is below the 10th percentile for newborns. If it is, the newborn will now be considered small for gestational age (SGA), the term used for pediatric care. In many hospitals, if the baby weighs more than 5 pounds and greater than 36 weeks' gestation, and little or no resuscitation treatment is needed, the baby will not need to go to the neonatal ICU. It can stay with the mother and be discharged with her when she leaves the hospital.

In the newborn period, the SGA infant is at risk for a number of complications. Difficulty getting enough oxygen may be present with significant prematurity. The baby may have difficulty maintaining its body temperature, and may need to stay on a warming bed or in an incubator. Low blood sugar is more common and IV glucose may need to be administered. If the baby has trouble sucking, a tube may need to be inserted through the mouth or nose into the stomach to infuse sufficient calories. All of these issues will need to be resolved before the baby can be discharged. This may take weeks depending on the degree of prematurity and growth lag. After discharge, catch-up growth occurs between 6 and 24 months of age, with 85% of SGA babies achieving a normal weight and height by age 2.[4] The baby's growth will be followed closely by the pediatrician, as those that do not grow appropriately will be at risk for short stature for life. Growth hormone may then be given in an effort to accelerate growth.

CASE STUDY #1

Carrie was at 27 weeks in her second pregnancy when she remarked to her physician that she felt smaller in this pregnancy than in the first. On examination, the uterus measured only 22 cm, 5 cm less than average. Carrie was taking nifedipine for her hypertension, but otherwise the pregnancy had been normal to date. Her genetic screening test had reported a risk of Down syndrome of less than 1 per 1,000, and her 20-week ultrasound had shown no fetal anomalies. Her physician ordered an ultrasound, and the measurements showed the head circumference (HC) at the 25th percentile, the femur length (FL) at the 15th percentile, and the abdominal circumference (AC) at the 6th percentile, with the overall EFW at the 12th percentile. The amniotic fluid volume was normal. A repeat ultrasound was scheduled for three weeks later, which showed that the HC was now at the 15th percentile, with the FL at the 10th percentile and the AC at the 5th percentile. The EFW was now at the 7th percentile. The amniotic fluid level was still normal, and a Doppler study of the umbilical artery was now elevated. A plan was made to start weekly fetal surveillance with NSTs and umbilical artery Dopplers, and these were initially normal. However, at 33 weeks the ultrasound now showed the AC less than the 3rd percentile, the EFW at the 5th percentile, the amniotic fluid level now low, and absent diastolic flow in the umbilical artery. Carrie was admitted to the hospital for a course of antenatal corticosteroids to advance fetal lung maturation, with twice-daily NSTs. Two days later, a labor induction was started, but the fetus began to demonstrate recurrent decelerations in the fetal heart rate. A cesarean delivery was performed, and a male infant was delivered weighing 3½ pounds (normal at this gestational age is 4½ to 5 pounds). The baby needed supplemental oxygen for three days and needed IV glucose to maintain his blood sugar level. A feeding tube was used for the first two weeks due to inadequate caloric intake, and he was able to maintain his body temperature after seven days in an incubator. He was ultimately discharged in good condition on day 24 of life, weighing 5 pounds. Carrie's recovery from her cesarean was normal.

CASE STUDY #2

In her third pregnancy, Noelle had her ultrasound at 20 weeks, when it was first suspected that her fetus was not growing appropriately. Measurements of the head and abdominal circumferences and femur length were symmetrically small and were 2–3 weeks behind. No other abnormalities or birth defects were identified. Serum screening was risk-reducing when performed at 12 weeks but did not exclude the possibility of a chromosomal abnormality. She had no medical issues that are risk factors for fetal growth restriction. In a search for the cause, blood tests were performed, with negative tests for antiphospholipid antibodies and recent infection with CMV and toxoplasmosis. An amniocentesis was performed *for genetic analyses, and significant abnormalities were found in genes known to be associated with stillbirth and growth restriction. Follow-up ultrasound three weeks later demonstrated that a stillbirth had occurred.*

SUMMARY

Fetal growth restriction can result from fetal conditions or inadequate delivery of nutrients to the fetus, which can lead to a deterioration in fetal well-being. There is little to be done to prevent or correct either of these situations. Rather, attention is turned to assessing the cause and when possible monitoring the fetal condition to prevent stillbirth. Some fetuses tolerate growth restriction due to the inadequate delivery of nutrients, and the pregnancy can be extended for many weeks, while others show signs of compromise, which requires delivery to avert an adverse outcome. With appropriate monitoring, most often the prognosis for the pregnancy is quite favorable, even if early delivery is necessary.

CHAPTER 19

CONGENITAL INFECTIONS

LIKE EVERYONE ELSE, pregnant women are exposed to bacteria and viruses in the environment. The hormones of pregnancy modify some elements of the immune system, but pregnant women do not appear to be more susceptible to infections than other people. It is not uncommon to contract colds, influenza, and stomach viruses while pregnant, and these rarely cause a pregnancy complication. However, there are other infectious agents that can cause major problems during pregnancy. In this chapter we will address some of them.

CYTOMEGALOVIRUS

Cytomegalovirus, or CMV, may be the most common virus you have never heard of. Most adults who get the virus are asymptomatic, although some get symptoms similar to those of the flu. As such, it is rarely tested for, so most people who have had it never know it. It can be more dangerous for immunocompromised people, such as those with HIV or a kidney transplant, but otherwise it is only a problem if you get it during pregnancy. In fact, it is the most common congenital infection that mothers pass to their fetuses, being found in approximately 1% of all newborns. Most of these infections are passed to the fetus through the placenta, which is known as vertical transmission, but the infection can also be acquired from the mother during delivery or through breastfeeding. When the mother contracts CMV for the first time (primary infection), she can develop fever, chills, muscle aches, enlarged lymph nodes, and liver inflammation, but again, most adults who are primarily infected with CMV are asymptomatic. Secondary infections can occur through reinfection or from reactivation of virus that lies dormant in the body. Transmission from person to person occurs via direct contact with infected blood, urine, saliva, or other bodily fluids. Children frequently acquire the virus in daycare settings, so women may be at higher risk in their second and subsequent pregnancies.

Most babies born with CMV are asymptomatic at birth, but those with severe complications may be affected with jaundice, low platelet counts, enlarged liver and spleen, and heart inflammation. Later manifestations may include hearing loss, vision issues, developmental and motor delay, and seizures. In general, the later in pregnancy a woman acquires CMV, the higher the chances of transmission to the fetus, but the milder the consequences. With infection in the first trimester, the risk of vertical transmission is lower, but of those fetuses that are affected the complications are more likely to be severe.

Since most people who acquire CMV are asymptomatic or have symptoms that mimic common viruses, women are rarely tested for CMV during pregnancy. In cases where maternal primary infection occurs in the first trimester and it is transmitted to the fetus, signs of severe complications may be seen on ultrasound in the second trimester, which may lead to the mother being tested. These signs could include calcifications in the brain and liver, excess fluid in the brain (hydrocephalus), fetal growth restriction, bright echoes in the intestines (echogenic bowel), and hydrops fetalis (discussed in chapter 20). When these signs are seen, the prognosis is poor, as stillbirth or the more severe complications mentioned above are likely to be seen after the baby is born. Other conditions can have some of these signs, so confirmation of the infection is usually recommended with amniocentesis and the finding of CMV DNA in the fluid. There are no treatments available to reduce the chances of vertical transmission or to lessen the effects of infection in the fetus. In situations where severe complications are likely, some women make the difficult decision to terminate the pregnancy if this option is available to them. When no signs of CMV are seen on ultrasound, CMV infection is only suspected if abnormalities are identified in the newborn period.

If a woman has a child in a daycare setting, there may be other children there who contract the infection. Sharing toys and being close to other children will put her child at risk of getting the virus and bringing it home. When you have a toddler at home, it is difficult not to be exposed to their bodily fluids while changing diapers or if they are sick. The best advice to avoid getting the infection during pregnancy is to practice good hand washing every time you are exposed to your child's body fluids, but avoidance still may not be possible. Nurses who are pregnant and working in an intensive care unit setting should avoid caring for patients infected with CMV if possible.

TOXOPLASMOSIS

Toxoplasmosis, often referred to as toxo, is an infection caused by a parasite acquired primarily by ingesting undercooked meat from an infected animal. It can also be acquired by contact with food contaminated by insects carrying the parasite, or by contact with the feces of infected cats. Indoor cats are rarely infected, and human infection can be avoided by not being the one who changes the litter box, wearing gloves when you do change it, and hand washing after.

Most people who get toxoplasmosis are asymptomatic, although some get fever, swollen lymph glands, malaise, joint pain, and swelling of the liver and spleen. Vertical transmission through the placenta to the fetus occurs only 10–15% of the time with first trimester infections, 25% of the time with second trimester infections, and more than 60% of the time with third trimester infections, but like CMV, the earlier in the pregnancy the fetus is infected, the more likely the disease will be severe.[1] Ultrasound findings sometimes seen with infected fetuses can be similar to CMV and include excess fluid, calcium deposits, and abscesses in the brain, an enlarged liver, fetal growth restriction, bright echoes in the intestines, and hydrops fetalis. Most infected newborns do not show signs of infection at birth, but may still develop vision impairment, hearing loss, and severe cognitive delay.

Unfortunately, current blood tests for susceptibility and immunity to toxoplasmosis are not particularly helpful because of many false positive results. As such, routine screening for all pregnant women is not recommended, and detecting cases of asymptomatic infection are not practical. For pregnant women who are symptomatic, or if abnormal findings on ultrasound suggest the possibility of toxo, the blood tests then can be helpful for the diagnosis, and there are treatments available that can be given during pregnancy. These medications do not prevent vertical transmission to the fetus, but they may reduce the severity of the disease. The best strategies for preventing toxo infections are to avoid eating raw or undercooked meat while pregnant, and washing vegetables and then your hands when preparing meals.

SYPHILIS

Syphilis is an infectious disease caused by a bacterium acquired through sexual activity. It starts as a painless sore and then is manifested by a rash. Subsequently, the infection becomes hidden without symptoms, but the patient is still infectious. The number of reported cases of syphilis in the United States was over 200,000 in 1950, but dropped significantly over the next 50 years, with less than 35,000 cases in the five years after 2000. But the number of cases in the United States rose more than fourfold since 2010, with over 207,000 cases reported in 2022.[2] This is a major public health concern not only for the serious complications that syphilis can cause in later life but also because pregnant women can transmit it to their fetuses. This is why all pregnant women should be tested for syphilis at the first prenatal visit, and higher-risk patients should be retested in the last month of pregnancy. Over 9,000 pregnant women are now diagnosed with syphilis in the United States annually.[3] If untreated for years, syphilis can lead to brain complications, heart disease, and damage to other internal organs.

If untreated during pregnancy, syphilis can cause serious complications in the fetus. These complications include fetal anemia, bone damage, an enlarged spleen, excess amniotic fluid, and hydrops fetalis. Many of these will be evident on ultrasound, along with an enlarged placenta. After delivery, the newborn can have a rash, jaundice, abnormal teeth, and meningitis, but ultimately can be found to have deafness, blindness, and intellectual disability. Approximately 40% of cases of untreated congenital syphilis end in stillbirth or death in the newborn period. Fortunately, syphilis is curable with penicillin. If treatment is provided to an infected individual during pregnancy, it can prevent transmission and lessen or prevent complications in the baby and the mom.

PARVOVIRUS B19

Parvovirus is another infection often spread by small children through respiratory secretions and saliva. When a child gets this virus, manifestations include a facial rash, sometimes followed by a rash on the body, fever, and joint pains, and is called "fifth disease."

Many adults with the infection are asymptomatic, but some also develop a body rash, fever, and joint pain. Most infections in both children and adults are benign, with a complete recovery within a week. Parvovirus testing is done through blood work for short- (IgM) and long-term (IgG) antibodies. If a person has only IgG antibodies, it is a sign that they have had a prior infection and are immune. Those with neither antibodies are susceptible. Once a person is infected, IgM antibodies are formed within 2–3 weeks of the exposure and last one or more months before IgG antibodies begin to form. More than half of reproductive-age women are IgG positive and, therefore, immune.

Most often parvovirus comes to light when a child develops a fever and rash and a pediatrician diagnoses "fifth disease." If the child's mother or another household member is pregnant, she should be tested for parvovirus antibodies. If she has IgG antibodies to the virus, there is no risk. If she is IgG antibody negative, there is a 50% chance that she will become infected and begin to form IgM antibodies within a few weeks. If this occurs, the risk of vertical transmission to the fetus is in the range of 20–30%. While most infected fetuses resolve the infection without complications, there is risk of miscarriage or stillbirth, with the risk of fetal loss being much lower in the second half of pregnancy. The risk of pregnancy loss is primarily within 10 weeks of maternal infection. If no complications have occurred by that time, most likely the fetus will have been unaffected by the virus.

One of the effects of the virus is to cause the fetus to stop making red bloods, and the fetus becomes progressively anemic. Once the blood count is extremely low, it results in heart failure and collection of fluid in the fetus (hydrops fetalis). Pregnant women who have antibody evidence of infection should be followed with ultrasound weekly for up to three months looking for hydrops. But they should also have Doppler assessment of blood flow of a brain artery each time, as described in chapter 25. If severe anemia develops, this measurement rises, often before hydrops sets in. The treatment for this is an intrauterine transfusion of blood, described in chapter 25 as well. This transfusion can be lifesaving for the fetus, but fortunately is not necessary very often.

ZIKA

The Zika virus first came to widespread public attention in 2015 after a large epidemic occurred in Brazil. The virus is spread by a particular species of mosquitos, and cases have been reported in almost half the countries in the world. However, the number of cases of Zika infection has declined significantly from 2017 to the present, and now only sporadic cases are reported to occur, primarily in South and Central America and the Caribbean, with only a handful of countries having more than 100 cases in all of 2023.

Most people infected with the Zika virus are asymptomatic or experience only mild symptoms. The concern is for infection during pregnancy, when vertical transmission to the fetus can occur. The virus causes birth defects in approximately 5% of babies born to women who contract Zika during pregnancy, and these can be quite serious, including brain and eye defects, developmental delay, hearing and vision problems, and seizures. There are no treatments for Zika that can prevent these complications in the fetus. However, these types of complications were mainly seen in tropical and subtropical locations, and are no longer a significant problem in these areas or elsewhere. There have been no confirmed Zika cases acquired in the United States since 2018.[4]

OTHER VIRUSES THAT CAN AFFECT PREGNANCY

There are a number of other viruses that can cause complications during pregnancy, but they are very uncommon. Rubella, also known as German measles, can cause major birth defects, especially when contracted in the first trimester. Since rubella vaccination in childhood has become the rule, infection during pregnancy is now rare in countries with large-scale immunization programs. Varicella, or chicken pox, can result in skin scarring of the fetus, eye disease, and limb malformations, but this infection is also now rarely seen during pregnancy in immunized populations. Coxsackievirus, which causes hand, foot, and mouth disease in children, is associated with a slightly increased risk of pregnancy complications such as fetal heart muscle dysfunction. There is no vaccine to prevent coxsackie infection. Immunity from prior infections or vaccines for these viruses are the best ways to limit the harmful effects. Occasional cases are seen in some immigrant populations and in the unvaccinated.

CASE STUDY #1

Mandy was at 12 weeks' gestation in her second pregnancy when she called her obstetrician's office to report that her 2-year-old had a rash and fever, and had been diagnosed with fifth disease. She was instructed to come to the office the next day for blood work. Parvovirus antibody levels were drawn and returned that she had neither IgG nor IgM, signifying that she was susceptible. She was instructed to return for repeat testing in three weeks, when test results now showed the presence of IgM antibodies, meaning that she had been infected even though she remained asymptomatic. A plan was made for her to return weekly for ultrasound examination for the next three months. The ultrasounds remained normal until 20 weeks, when the Doppler study of the fetal middle cerebral artery was quite elevated. It was explained that most likely the fetus was now severely anemic and would likely develop hydrops fetalis if not transfused. She agreed to a transfusion procedure the next day, and a needle was inserted into her uterus through her abdomen under ultrasound guidance, directly into a vein in the umbilical cord. Blood was drawn and analyzed showing that the fetus had lost more than two-thirds of its blood cells, and a transfusion was initiated. The fetus tolerated the procedure, with the blood count at the end of the procedure normal for a fetus at this gestational age. Follow-up ultrasounds showed that the fetus continued in good condition without signs of anemia, and a healthy male infant was delivered at term.

CASE STUDY #2

Kiko was at 20 weeks in her third pregnancy when an ultrasound found multiple abnormalities. These included fetal growth restriction, hydrocephalus, and echogenic bowel. Further, calcifications were noted in the brain and in the liver. These findings suggested the presence of congenital infection. Kiko had no recollection of a viral illness earlier in the pregnancy, but both of her children were in daycare. Blood work was drawn for CMV and toxo testing—IgG and IgM were both positive for CMV, and both negative for toxo. This could either be due to a recent CMV infection or a past CMV infection with persistent IgM. An amniocentesis was performed, and CMV DNA was detected, confirming the diagnosis of fetal infection. Kiko and her partner were counseled regarding the possible effects of CMV on a child, and that in her case the effects would likely be severe given the ultrasound findings. This pregnancy was very much desired by this couple, but they had strong feelings that having a child with severe brain damage was not something they wanted for their family. Ultimately, they decided to terminate the pregnancy.

SUMMARY

Bacteria, viruses, and parasites are part of the environment that we live in. A healthy immune system helps to prevent and fight these infections, so most common infections do not present major risks. However, there are some infections that can cause major complications in pregnancy, and most viruses do not have a treatment that can change the course of the illness or prevent complications. The first step is to identify the cause of an infection, and then to assess whether it puts the fetus at risk. Ultrasound is often the best modality for assessment of the effects on the fetus, but some adverse consequences will not be evident until after birth or even years later. The best approach to infection prevention is immunity from prior exposure or vaccination.

CHAPTER 20

HYDROPS FETALIS

SOME OF THE CONDITIONS described in this book list hydrops fetalis as a possible result of the complication. "Hydrops fetalis" is a term used to describe collections of excess fluid within two or more body cavities of the fetus. This fluid can collect in the abdomen, around the heart and lungs, in the skin, and in the amniotic cavity. The causes are varied, but they include cardiac anomalies or arrhythmias, heart failure, fetal infections, structural anomalies, genetic abnormalities, and fetal anemia. Hydrops is often a sign of the progression of the condition, with fetal death the likely outcome. Even if the baby is delivered, the mortality rate is high, as fluid in the chest can obstruct lung expansion and function, and the heart and other organs may be compromised as well.

CAUSES OF HYDROPS FETALIS

There is a long list of conditions that can lead to hydrops, and these are listed in box 20.1. They include infections, genetic syndromes, severe anemia, cardiac arrhythmias, structural defects, blood disorders, and tumors. It can also be seen in identical twin pregnancies when twin-to-twin transfusion syndrome develops (chapter 27).

BOX 20.1 CONDITIONS THAT CAN LEAD TO HYDROPS FETALIS

- Blood group incompatibility
- Fetal anemia
- Cardiac
  - Tachycardia
  - Myocarditis
  - Congenital heart defects
- Structural defects
  - Pulmonary airway malformations
  - Dwarfism
- Infections
  - Cytomegalovirus
  - Toxoplasmosis
  - Syphilis
  - Parvovirus
- Genetic disorders
  - Chromosomal abnormalities—Turner, Down syndrome
  - Alpha thalassemia
  - Metabolic disorders—Niemann-Pick disease, Gaucher disease
- Tumors—teratomas
- Twin-to-twin transfusion syndrome

Sometimes the excess fluid that collects is a result of heart failure due to one of these conditions, poor lymphatic drainage of body cavities, or reduced protein in the blood allowing fluid to leak out of the circulation.

Causes of hydrops are often divided into immune and nonimmune hydrops. Immune hydrops, discussed in more depth in chapter 25, is caused by blood group incompatibility between the fetus and the mother, with maternal antibodies crossing into the fetal circulation through the placenta and attacking and destroying fetal red blood cells. The resulting anemia leads to increased cardiac output in an effort to deliver more oxygen to the tissues with few oxygen-carrying red cells. The heart eventually cannot keep up and heart failure ensues. All other causes are referred to as nonimmune hydrops.

EVALUATION OF HYDROPS FETALIS

Hydrops is diagnosed by ultrasound with the findings of excess fluid in any two of the following: abdominal cavity (ascites), amniotic sac (polyhydramnios), chest (pleural effusion), sac around the heart (pericardial effusion), or under the skin. When hydrops is identified, an investigation for the cause is then undertaken. This evaluation includes a detailed ultrasound looking for any structural abnormalities associated with hydrops (cardiac defects, masses in the chest, and tumors), heart rate abnormalities, and calcifications in the brain, liver, or intestines. Ultrasound of the middle cerebral artery (MCA) in the brain using Doppler can determine whether severe fetal anemia is present. Blood work is done to test for blood group incompatibility and infections. If not already done, genetic testing is offered, looking for genetic causes. If none of these tests reveal an explanation, diagnosis may need to await further evaluation after delivery. Alternatively, fetal blood can be obtained for testing by inserting a needle through the mother's abdomen into the umbilical cord. Efforts to reveal the cause of hydrops is important in giving the parents a better idea of the prognosis, and the chances of recurrence in a future pregnancy.

TREATMENTS FOR HYDROPS FETALIS

There are few causes of hydrops for which treatment can improve the prognosis. If fetal anemia is detected, an intrauterine transfusion can correct the anemia with complete resolution of hydrops. Medications to control the fetal heart rate can be beneficial if the cause is tachycardia. If twin-to-twin transfusion syndrome is present, laser surgery may be able to reverse the process and allow the pregnancy to continue. But otherwise treatment is usually not helpful, and alternatives to continuing the pregnancy might need to be discussed if the mother decides not to carry the pregnancy to term. You might think that inserting a needle into the body cavity and removing the excess fluid would help. However, this is rarely the case, as the fluid routinely re-collects in that space when the underlying cause is not corrected.

CASE STUDY #1

Serita was at 20 weeks in her second pregnancy when she came for her scheduled ultrasound appointment. Her first pregnancy was uneventful and delivered at term without complications. During the ultrasound it was revealed that the baby had an enlarged liver, and excess fluid in the abdominal cavity and chest, with skin edema and polyhydramnios as well. There were no signs of structural abnormalities or calcifications, and the heart rate was in the normal range. Doppler studies of the middle cerebral artery were not indicative of fetal anemia. The concerning nature of the condition was discussed with Serita and her partner, along with a plan for further investigation. Review of her records showed a blood type of A positive with no antibodies that could attack fetal red blood cells, but Serita had previously declined genetic testing. After counseling that the most likely causes of the hydrops now were infection and genetic syndromes, she agreed to testing for both. Blood for antibody testing showed no sign of recent infection with CMV, toxoplasmosis, or parvovirus, and cell-free DNA testing showed a very low risk of Down syndrome. However, the carrier screen showed that she was a carrier for Gaucher disease, a disorder which can lead to enlargement of the liver, brain dysfunction, and poor growth. Her partner was subsequently tested and he was also a carrier for this disease. Fetal blood sampling was suggested as a means to confirm the diagnosis, and results returned that indeed the fetus had inherited both abnormal genes for Gaucher disease. At 24 weeks, Serita noted that she no longer felt the baby moving, and fetal death was confirmed by ultrasound. Labor was induced, and she delivered a stillborn fetus with hydrops.

Serita and her partner were counseled that in the future each time they conceived there would be a 25% risk of the fetus being affected with this disease. Six months after the last delivery, Serita underwent IVF with genetic testing of the ten embryos that were obtained. One of the seven embryos without the mutation for Gaucher was implanted successfully, and she went on to have a normal pregnancy. She gave birth to a healthy female infant.

CASE STUDY #2

Grace had a normal pregnancy until 30 weeks, when she reported decreased fetal movement to her physician. An ultrasound was ordered and no anomalies were detected, but pericardial and pleural effusions were present with some excess fluid in the abdomen noted, along with a biophysical profile score that was reassuring. A fetal cardiac echo was obtained the next day, showing no cardiac *defects but decreased contractility of the ventricular walls suggesting mild to moderate heart failure. Review of prior testing revealed a very low risk of chromosomal abnormality based on cell-free DNA testing, blood type O positive with a negative antibody screen, and a normal carrier screen result. Blood was sent for CMV and toxo testing, and both returned IgM negative and IgG positive, inconsistent with recent infection. Amniocentesis was performed, and coxsackievirus was detected in the amniotic fluid. Grace stated that one of her children was diagnosed with hand, foot, and mouth disease three weeks previously (caused by coxsackievirus), but she had not had any symptoms of a viral illness.*

Grace's pregnancy was followed closely with fetal surveillance three times a week, which remained reassuring. Cardiac echoes were repeated twice weekly and were without signs of worsening hydrops or further deterioration in heart function. Two weeks after her initial diagnosis, the excess fluid in the abdominal cavity had resolved, as had the pleural effusion. In another week, the pericardial effusion had also resolved, and ventricular contractility was improved. At 37 weeks, Grace went into spontaneous labor and delivered a female infant with no apparent signs of distress. A cardiac echo in the nursery showed normal heart function. A diagnosis of fetal coxsackievirus infection with heart inflammation which had resolved spontaneously was made, and Grace was able to take home a healthy baby girl.

SUMMARY

Finding hydrops fetalis on an ultrasound places the pregnancy in serious jeopardy. There is a wide range of diseases and conditions that can result in hydrops, so a thorough investigation is necessary to identify the cause. In a few cases, treatment can be helpful, and in others the hydrops will resolve on its own. Immune hydrops due to blood group incompatibility can be correctible with a fetal blood transfusion, but non-immune hydrops is most often uncorrectable, with a very high rate of stillbirth or neonatal death. Identifying the cause of hydrops is important to give the parents an accurate prognosis, an idea of its chance of recurrence in future pregnancies, and options to improve the chances of success in those future pregnancies.

PART V

PREGNANCY CONDITIONS

CHAPTER 21

PRETERM BIRTH

PRETERM BIRTH CONTINUES to be one of the major problems in obstetrics, and its prevention and treatment have eluded researchers for decades. About 1 in 10 infants born in the United States is born before 37 weeks, which is considered full term for a single gestation, one of the highest rates in the developed world. Behind only birth defects, prematurity is the second leading cause of infant mortality. An estimate of the lifetime societal cost related to preterm birth in the United States in 2016 was over $25 billion annually, and this cost goes up every year.[1] And there is significant variation by race, with the rate of preterm birth almost 50% higher among African Americans than among White Americans.

Preterm birth is divided by degree of prematurity. Late preterm infants are born between 34 and 36 weeks of pregnancy, moderately preterm infants are born between 32 and 34 weeks, very preterm babies are born between 25 and 32 weeks, and extremely preterm infants at less than 25 weeks' gestation. Preterm births can also be divided into those that are spontaneous (including premature labor and premature rupture of membranes) and those that are indicated, where a decision is made to deliver to benefit the mother or the baby.

The earlier the infant is born, the higher the risk of complications. These risks to the baby include respiratory distress syndrome (RDS), intracranial hemorrhage potentially leading to cerebral palsy, infections, bowel complications, and death. For babies born before 28 weeks, the risk of death or cerebral palsy is 10% or higher.[2]

RISK FACTORS FOR PRETERM BIRTH

Preterm delivery in an earlier pregnancy is the most common risk factor for preterm birth, with a recurrence risk of 20%. Multiple gestation is also a leading cause of preterm birth, with more than 50% of twins and 90% of triplets born before 37 completed weeks. This also means that multiple gestations have increased risk of delivering very preterm and extremely preterm. Although 2–3% of all births are multiple gestations, twins and triplets routinely make up 15–20% of babies in neonatal intensive care units (NICUs) because of issues related to prematurity.[3] Other risk factors for spontaneous preterm delivery include uterine anomalies, cervical insufficiency, certain fetal anomalies, short interval between pregnancies, smoking, advanced maternal age, in vitro fertilization, and certain infections. The development of preeclampsia is the most common pregnancy complication leading to an indicated preterm delivery, but other causes include fetal growth restriction, placenta previa, and placental abruption.

CONSEQUENCES OF PRETERM BIRTH

As stated previously, the earlier a baby is born, the higher the risks of complications. Babies born between 34 and 36 weeks (late preterm) make up 8% of all births, and 74% of all preterm births.[4] Most babies born in this range have few concerning issues, but these could include low blood sugar, inability to maintain body temperature, jaundice, and a short-term need for oxygen supplementation, especially if the mother did not receive a course of steroids prior to delivery. These tend to be short-term issues, lasting only a few days, and rarely have any long-term health implications, but they still may require admission to the NICU. Low blood sugar may require bottle feeding or an IV with glucose for a day or two, and babies having trouble with their body temperature regulation may need to be in an incubator or under a heat lamp. Jaundice is usually treated with UV lights for a short period of time. Concerns have been raised by studies showing that babies born between 34 and 36 weeks are more likely than their term counterparts to develop cognitive delays, autism, and attention deficit hyperactivity disorder (ADHD).[5] The mortality rate and rate of cerebral palsy for babies born in this gestational age range are both less than 1%, but still 3–6 times higher than babies born at 37 weeks or after.[6]

Moderately preterm infants have higher levels of risk of the issues discussed for late preterm infants, and also a few other risks. One of these risks is feeding difficulties, which could require placement of a tube through the nose or mouth into the stomach to deliver milk and other nutrients. RDS rates for this group are 20%, and can on occasion require a tube placed through the nose or mouth to deliver oxygen.[7] The mortality rate for babies born in this gestational age window was sixfold higher than for term infants.

Very preterm births account for less than 2% of all live births in the United States, but account for more than 50% of infant deaths.[8] Yet, with medical advances over the last few decades, survival rates range from roughly 75% at 25 weeks to better than 95% at 32 weeks.[9] Complications are much more common for infants born in this gestational age range, and often more worrisome. These include bleeding in the brain, bowel complications, heart issues, long-term oxygen dependence, and damage to the eyes (ROP, or retinopathy of prematurity). Longer-term health issues are also more common, and these include development of chronic lung disease, cerebral palsy, and blindness.

Babies born extremely prematurely are now being resuscitated more frequently, as the survival rates for this group have increased. The survival to discharge rates for babies born at weeks 22, 23, and 24 between 2013 and 2018 were 28%, 54%, and 70%, respectively.[10] Major complications were encountered routinely, with rates ranging from 98–100% for needing a ventilator, 6–9% requiring surgery for necrotizing enterocolitis (NEC), a bowel injury, 25–38% for bleeding in the brain, 31–38% for severe ROP, and 13–15% for needing surgery for a heart problem. For those babies that survived, average hospital stays were four to five months. Only 10%, 18%, and 23% of babies born at 22, 23, and 24 weeks survived with no or mild neurodevelopmental impairment.[11]

DIAGNOSIS AND MANAGEMENT OF PREMATURE LABOR

Spontaneous premature labor is diagnosed when, before 37 weeks, a mother develops regular painful contractions which lead to progressive cervical dilation. The presence of contractions alone are not sufficient to make this diagnosis. There are times when a patient with contractions shows some degree of cervical dilation, but the dilation does not progress to delivery or the contractions abate. Some degree of patience is necessary in observing the contractions to decide that delivery is inevitable, and this is usually when the dilation of the cervix is greater than 4 cm.

Premature rupture of membranes (also known as PROM and more commonly as when a woman's water breaks) is when a break occurs in the sac around the baby containing the amniotic fluid. The woman usually experiences a gush of fluid, and PROM can usually be distinguished from leaking urine by noting repetitive loss of fluid. PROM can occur before a patient experiences any labor symptoms. On occasion, the amount of fluid lost is very small, which can lead to some ambiguity in the diagnosis. Tests can be run on the fluid coming from the cervix to determine that it is indeed amniotic fluid. With PROM, the barrier between the fetal environment and the vagina is lost, which can lead to bacteria ascending from the vagina into the uterus and causing a serious infection called chorioamnionitis (or amnionitis), or it can initiate the process of labor. In cases where the membranes have broken, delivery should only be delayed under medical supervision.

Over the years, many medications have been tried to treat premature labor and prevent early delivery. Some may slow contractions and delay delivery by a few days. But none of these agents have been found to lengthen pregnancy for more than a few days, and none are FDA approved for this indication. Activity may stimulate contractions during the pregnancy, but bed rest has not been shown to prolong pregnancy. What is important is giving steroids to the mother when preterm delivery appears likely within a week, whether due to premature labor, premature rupture of membranes, or some reason for an indicated delivery. Steroids given to the mother prior to delivery improve neonatal lung function, and they reduce the risks of brain hemorrhage, bowel complications, and neonatal death. The steroid most used currently is betamethasone, given as a course of two injections 24 hours apart. It is thought to have some benefit within 12 hours of the first dose, with full efficacy at 48 hours. However, this efficacy is thought to diminish after about a week. There is also evidence to support repeating this course of steroids one time for a mother who appears to be at risk of delivery within 7 days, if the prior course was administered more than 14 days previously and the gestational age is still less than 34 weeks.[12] Although magnesium sulfate and indomethacin have not been shown to provide significant pregnancy prolongation, they may be helpful in slowing contractions and delaying delivery by hours to days to allow time for the steroids to benefit the fetus.

A more recent controversy has arisen regarding the benefits of the hormone progesterone in prevention of preterm birth. A landmark research study published in 2003 randomized patients with a prior preterm birth to weekly progesterone injections versus placebo starting before 20 weeks, and showed a significant reduction in repeat preterm delivery, especially prior to 32 weeks.[13] Based on this study, a number of organizations, including the American College of Obstetricians and Gynecologists as well as the March of Dimes, advocated for the routine use of this hormone for patients with prior preterm birth. The FDA did approve progesterone for this indication under the condition that a confirmatory study be conducted in the near future. This second study was published in 2019, and showed a contradictory result—no benefit in preventing preterm birth or reducing infant deaths.[14] In 2023, the FDA voted to remove the approval for this medication, and it is no longer advocated for this indication. Progesterone suppositories may still be used as a treatment option for a patient with a history of preterm delivery if her cervix is found to be short in the mid-trimester.

CASE STUDY #1

Morgan was 28 weeks pregnant when she called her physician's office to report having uterine tightening beginning early that morning. The pregnancy had been uncomplicated to that point, and the fetus was active. The tightening was now every 7–10 minutes and getting more regular over the previous two hours. She denied any leaking fluid or bleeding. She was told to come to the hospital, where the monitor revealed contractions every 5–6 minutes with a normal fetal heart rate pattern, and on pelvic exam the cervix was only 1.5 cm long (normal 3–5 cm) and 2 cm dilated. She was admitted for observation and intravenous fluids were administered. When the contractions got stronger and more frequent, her cervix was now 3 cm dilated and she was given an injection of betamethasone and started on a 48-hour course of indomethacin in an effort to slow contractions. Repeat cervical examinations showed no further dilation, and a second dose of betamethasone was given 24 hours later. On day two after admission, contractions seemed less frequent and were milder, and cervical dilation had not progressed. Morgan was discharged for follow-up in the office in one week. At 31 weeks she again came to the hospital for more frequent contractions and was now found to be 4 cm dilated with regular contractions every four minutes. A repeat course of betamethasone was started as was another course of indomethacin. The next morning she reported leaking fluid, and rupture of membranes was confirmed on examination. The contractions then became more intense and she was given an epidural for pain relief. She delivered a girl named Megan vaginally three hours later weighing 3 pounds, 13 ounces, and Megan was taken to the NICU. The infant had mild respiratory distress syndrome requiring oxygen, but no evidence of an intracranial hemorrhage. After four days Megan was able to breathe normally on room air, and feeding with breast milk was initiated through a feeding tube. Megan grew progressively and was discharged doing well after five weeks in the ICU. She continues to develop normally.

CASE STUDY #2

Connie was 30 weeks pregnant when she noticed a large gush of clear fluid from her vagina. The pregnancy to this point had been uneventful. When she arrived at the hospital, rupture of membranes was confirmed, and ultrasound revealed that the fetus was in breech position with very little fluid around it. Only occasional contractions were seen on the monitor, and the fetal heart rate pattern was reassuring. A betamethasone injection was administered, and she was admitted to the hospital. It was explained to her that she should remain in the hospital for frequent monitoring, and that if labor began or infection set in she would need to be delivered. If she was still undelivered at 34 weeks, she would be delivered then, as at that point the risks for the infant of prematurity would be lower than the risk of continuing the pregnancy. Fetal heart rate monitoring was performed three times a week and remained reassuring; no fever or other signs of infection developed. She continued to leak fluid daily, and she received a second course of betamethasone at 32 weeks.

At 33 weeks, Connie experienced the onset of abdominal pain and noted that blood was now coming from her vagina. Fetal monitoring showed contractions every two minutes with decelerations of the fetal heart rate. A diagnosis of placental separation (abruption) was made, a known complication of PROM. She was rushed to the operating room, and an emergency cesarean was performed under general anesthesia. The newborn girl was transferred to the NICU before the cesarean was completed. An abruption was confirmed during the operation, where 50% of the placenta appeared to have detached from the uterine wall prior to delivery. Connie had no complications from the procedure, and after four hours was able to visit her daughter in the NICU. The infant had mild RDS, needing supplemental oxygen for only two days, and was discharged three weeks later doing well.

SUMMARY

Preterm birth continues to be the most common complication of pregnancy, and it accounts for a significant portion of neonatal complications and deaths. Preterm deliveries often result in stays in the NICU and additional treatment for the baby may be required. In addition, developmental delays might appear, especially for babies born extremely prematurely. The earlier in the pregnancy a baby is born, the more at risk they are for medical and developmental complications. There are no medications available that can prevent or stop premature labor or premature rupture of membranes, but when preterm birth appears likely, administration of steroids can reduce neonatal complications.

CHAPTER 22

PREECLAMPSIA

PREECLAMPSIA IS A CONDITION unique to pregnancy and is characterized by hypertension in association with swelling in the legs and protein loss in the urine. It is second in frequency only to premature birth among all complications, affecting more than 5% of pregnancies in the United States.[1] Preeclampsia is a leading cause of maternal mortality worldwide; timely diagnosis and treatment are the keys to preventing severe complications and deaths of both mother and child. Despite intensive research over decades, the cause of preeclampsia has yet to be determined, which has hindered efforts at prevention.

DEFINITIONS

As discussed in chapter 6, there are a number of conditions involving high blood pressure during pregnancy and, grouped together, they constitute the hypertensive disorders of pregnancy (HDP). These include chronic hypertension, gestational hypertension, preeclampsia, HELLP syndrome, and eclampsia. Chronic hypertension is often recognized in a patient prior to pregnancy, but if the hypertension is first noted in the first half of pregnancy, it is also considered chronic hypertension. Preeclampsia entails the development of hypertension in the second half of pregnancy, associated with protein in the urine (proteinuria), increased leg swelling, or both. Blood pressure elevation first identified in the second half of pregnancy is termed gestational hypertension if it does not have the other criteria that are present in preeclampsia, and the hypertension is expected to resolve after pregnancy. "Eclampsia" is the term used when pregnant patients with any form of hypertension develop one or more seizures. According to the Centers for Disease Control, over 15% of women giving birth in 2019 had an HDP, a percentage that has increased over the past ten years.[2]

The dilemma that arises is that patients often do not fit neatly into one category. Patients with gestational hypertension may develop proteinuria weeks after becoming hypertensive, so they are now considered to have preeclampsia. The hypertension in patients with gestation hypertension may not resolve after delivery, making it likely that chronic hypertension was the diagnosis all along. At least 10% of patients with preeclampsia do not develop proteinuria,[3] though they may have other signs (such as certain laboratory tests) that make the diagnosis likely. And patients with chronic hypertension are considered to have superimposed preeclampsia if in the second half of pregnancy the hypertension accelerates or they develop new or increased proteinuria. The development of proteinuria with hypertension is the best indicator that preeclampsia is present, and new onset seizures associated with hypertension confirm the diagnosis of eclampsia. Because there can be difficulty distinguishing between preeclampsia and gestation hypertension, the term "pregnancy induced hypertension" is sometimes used when either is present.

HELLP syndrome is a condition where significant abnormalities are present in a number of laboratory tests. These include hemolysis (H), elevated liver (EL) enzyme readings, and low platelets (LP). Hemolysis is the breakdown of red blood cells, elevated liver enzymes are a sign of liver injury, and low platelets can lead to bleeding complications. HELLP syndrome was originally described as developing in some patients who already were diagnosed with preeclampsia, but some patients demonstrate these laboratory abnormalities without hypertension. Even without elevations in blood pressure, HELLP syndrome is included as HDP.

Preeclampsia is characterized as mild or severe. Criteria that denote severe preeclampsia include blood pressure over 160/110 on more than one occasion more than four hours apart, development of pulmonary edema, laboratory values with elevated liver enzymes, low platelets, or rising creatinine, or the development of symptoms including persistent headache unresponsive to medication, or vision disturbances such as blurred vision. If none of these are present, preeclampsia is considered to be mild.

The reason to be concerned about preeclampsia is that it is a major cause of severe maternal complications and mortality for the mother, and premature birth for the baby. Among mothers who die during the delivery hospitalization, over 30% have an HDP.[4] Preeclampsia can lead to stroke, kidney failure, liver rupture, internal bleeding, and blindness. It can also lead to poor placental function, fetal growth restriction, placental detachment (abruption), and stillbirth. There is no cure for preeclampsia other than delivery, from which the vast majority of women recover completely. Delivery is therefore often performed before these serious complications can arise for the mother, but early delivery can lead to complications of prematurity for the newborn. Discussing options for delaying a delivery is advised, but delaying too long can result in worse outcomes for both the mother and the child.

Pregnancy-associated hypertension contributes significantly to the racial disparities in maternal complications and mortality. The incidence of preeclampsia is 50–100% higher in Black women, rates of severe complications are 50% higher, and the maternal mortality rate is almost threefold higher than in White women.[5] Higher rates of chronic diseases in the Black population that are risk factors for preeclampsia explain some of the disparity, but socioeconomic status, stress, and access to care likely play a role as well.[4] Black women and their caregivers should be aware of this disparity and take steps to recognize and treat preeclampsia and its complications before they become more severe.

RISK FACTORS FOR PREECLAMPSIA

There are many known risk factors for the development of preeclampsia. The ones placing you at highest risk include preeclampsia in a prior pregnancy, chronic hypertension, multiple gestation, diabetes, autoimmune disease, and kidney disease. Factors placing you at moderate risk include first pregnancy, obesity, mother or sister with preeclampsia, maternal age 35 or older, and being of Black race. More recent evidence suggests that IVF pregnancies are also at moderate risk independent of other factors. There are a number of risk calculators available that physicians can use to determine your level of risk, but most involve using tests that are not routinely performed, and their lack of accuracy limit their usefulness. According to the US Prevent Services Task Force, women at high risk for preeclampsia and those with two or more moderate risk factors based on the above criteria should begin taking a single low-dose aspirin tablet (81 mg) daily by the end of the first trimester to lower their risk, though you should discuss with your doctor before taking any medication.[6]

EVALUATION OF THE PATIENT WITH PREECLAMPSIA

When a patient in the second half of pregnancy has elevated blood pressure for the first time, the possibility of preeclampsia should be considered. The diagnosis of preeclampsia should await the finding of at least one more elevated blood pressure reading at least four hours later, but the evaluation can begin sooner than that. It will include assessment of the mother to determine whether she has any of the criteria for severe preeclampsia as well as an assessment of fetal well-being. The evaluation starts by asking about symptoms including headache, swelling, difficulty breathing, vision changes, and abdominal pain. Laboratory tests will include a red blood cell and platelet count, liver enzyme levels, creatinine level, and measurement of protein in the urine. An ultrasound examination of the fetus will be performed, if not already done recently, to assess fetal growth. Monitoring of the fetal heart rate will ensure that the fetus is currently stable. This evaluation will determine whether the patient is stable enough to be sent home or should be monitored in the hospital. In general, the condition worsens over time, so continued evaluation is an important part of management.

MANAGEMENT OF PREECLAMPSIA

When a diagnosis of preeclampsia is made, management depends on whether it is mild or severe, and the gestational age. If the pregnancy has reached 37 weeks, delivery is indicated whether mild or severe, because the risk at this stage of the condition worsening with waiting is greater than the risk of prematurity for the baby. If the condition is mild and the gestational age is fewer than 37 weeks, allowing the pregnancy to continue does run the risk that severe criteria will develop, but in most instances this risk is thought to be lower than the risks of prematurity for the fetus as long as both mother and fetus are stable. If prolonging the pregnancy is chosen, the evaluation outlined above and tests of fetal well-being (NST, BPP) are repeated at regular intervals. If other complications such as fetal growth restriction are also present, the plan may be modified.

If the patient meets severe criteria, delivery is indicated if the pregnancy has reached 34 weeks of gestation. The risks of severe complications from preeclampsia at this point outweigh the risks of prematurity for the newborn. Before 34 weeks, trying to extend the pregnancy may be an option if the only severe criterion is blood pressure. Blood pressure medication can be started or increased to lower the pressure and keep the mother safe, and frequent monitoring would be indicated. However, if concerning symptoms of unrelenting headache, severe upper abdomen pain, or difficulty breathing are present, or laboratory findings of elevated liver enzymes or low platelets develop, the risks for the mother are too great and delivery is recommended. Even at very early gestational ages, the fetus is likely better off being delivered if the mother's condition is deteriorating. Magnesium sulfate is given by IV during labor to reduce the risk of having an eclamptic seizure.

As mentioned previously, delivery is the only treatment that will resolve preeclampsia. It may take days for the sicker patients to recover completely, and the sickest patients may take even longer. Management after delivery involves controlling the blood pressure while the preeclampsia resolves itself. Blood pressure can increase again during the first two weeks after delivery, so monitoring the pressure after hospital discharge is important.

It is now recognized that having preeclampsia puts women at increased risk for developing heart disease, high blood pressure, and stroke later in life.[7] While seeking medical care after pregnancy, women should notify their primary care provider of their history of preeclampsia, as this will influence how their health is monitored for the rest of their lives. Your risk of developing these problems can be lowered with lifestyle changes, including stopping smoking and maintaining a healthy weight, and medications if you develop high blood pressure or elevated levels of cholesterol.

CASE STUDY #1

Katy's first pregnancy was complicated by preeclampsia, which was diagnosed at 37 weeks' gestation. She was induced the following day and delivered vaginally a 7-pound girl without complication. Her elevated blood pressure resolved within 24 hours of delivery, and she had no further issues with hypertension after discharge. Because of this history and her age of 38, Katy started taking a low-dose aspirin tablet in her next pregnancy at 12 weeks of gestation in an effort to lower the risk of preeclampsia recurrence. However, at 31 weeks she was noted to have a blood pressure of 150/100 and a moderate amount of protein in her urine. She denied any symptoms of severe preeclampsia, and laboratory tests revealed normal levels of platelets and liver enzymes. Ultrasound revealed that the baby's weight was below the 10th percentile, consistent with growth restriction. She was admitted to the hospital for closer monitoring and NST tests three times a week. Steroids were initiated in an effort to accelerate fetal lung maturation in the event of early delivery.

Two days after admission, Katy was noted to have multiple blood pressure readings above 160/110, signifying that her preeclampsia was now severe. Nifedipine, a medication used to control hypertension, was started to lower her blood pressure, and it stabilized in the 140s/90s range. At 33 weeks, her platelet count decreased from 130,000 on admission to 85,000, and her liver enzyme levels were now more than twice the upper limit of the normal range. Because of these abnormalities, a decision was made to induce her labor. During the labor she again had multiple blood pressure readings above 160/110, and she was given intravenous medication to lower her pressure. Magnesium sulfate was administered through her IV as well. She delivered vaginally, and the baby girl was taken to the neonatal ICU for care. The baby had signs of immature lung function, and needed supplemental oxygen for three days but no longer. She did well after that and was discharged three weeks after delivery weighing 4½ pounds.

Katy was discharged on nifedipine with instructions to take her blood pressure three times a day. A week after discharge she reported multiple readings above 160/110, and was instructed to increase her nifedipine dose. After this, she no longer had readings that high. Four weeks after delivery her blood pressures were all in the normal range. She was instructed to stop her medication, and the pressure remained in the normal range. Katy was advised that if she were to conceive again, she would be at even higher risk for a recurrence of her preeclampsia, and was told that she should share her diagnosis of preeclampsia with her primary care provider.

CASE STUDY #2

Cassandra was at 28 weeks' gestation in her first pregnancy when she presented to the emergency room with nausea and vomiting and a severe headache. While she was undergoing evaluation, she had a seizure. Magnesium sulfate was administered and no more seizures occurred. She had no history of hypertension, kidney disease, or seizures, and pregnancy to this point had been normal. Fetal monitoring was initiated, and showed a normal fetal heart rate with occasional decelerations. Laboratory tests were conducted, showing anemia, markedly elevated liver enzyme levels, and a platelet count of 55,000 (normal being over 100,000), with the highest reading for proteinuria. A diagnosis of eclampsia with HELLP syndrome was made, and preparations were begun for delivery. A primary cesarean was performed under general anesthesia, and a baby boy weighing only 2 pounds was delivered and transferred to the neonatal ICU intubated. The cesarean was completed and Cassandra was transferred to the maternal ICU for monitoring. Multiple medications were needed to control her blood pressure over the first 48 hours, and her laboratory values slowly corrected. However, bleeding developed under the skin of her abdomen due to her low platelet count and the cesarean incision opened. The incision needed frequent dressing changes, and began to close slowly on its own. She was eventually discharged on day six after delivery taking two blood pressure medications, and arrangements were made for a visiting nurse to provide home dressing changes while the incision was open. Over the next few weeks, the incision closed completely, and her blood pressure was back to her pre-pregnancy level on no medications by six weeks. The infant had multiple complications over the first two weeks, including respiratory distress and infection, but ultimately was stabilized without needing supplemental oxygen after three weeks. The infant was discharged after a two-month hospitalization, weighing just over 5 pounds, but at age 2 was showing signs of developmental delay.

SUMMARY

Preeclampsia is a common complication of pregnancy with many risk factors; it is also the most dangerous of the disorders of blood pressure that can present during pregnancy. Severe complications can develop, with maternal mortality a possibility if not monitored closely and treated aggressively. Patients with multiple risk factors, or those with one major risk factor, should take low-dose aspirin under a doctor's supervision during the pregnancy to lower the risk of it developing. If preeclampsia does develop, an evaluation is performed to determine whether it is mild or severe, and whether delivery is indicated for the well-being of the mother or baby. If the pregnancy is at term, delivery is indicated. If the diagnosis comes preterm but is mild, the preeclampsia is monitored for signs of severity and the baby can be carried to term if complications do not develop. Delivery is indicated if the mother develops severe preeclampsia, but attempts at delaying the delivery until 34 weeks may be possible if the mother and fetus are stable. Delivery resolves preeclampsia, if not immediately, then shortly thereafter, but the decision to deliver is made based on weighing the risks to the mother of prolonging the pregnancy versus the risks of premature delivery for the fetus. With appropriate care, most women recover completely after delivery, and their newborns do well with modern care for premature infants. Women who have had preeclampsia should be aware that they are at increased risk for hypertension, heart disease, and stroke later in life.

CHAPTER 23

PLACENTAL ABNORMALITIES

THE PLACENTA IS AN ORGAN of the fetus which serves many vital purposes for the pregnancy. It transports oxygen and vital nutrients from the mother's system into that of the fetus, produces hormones which the fetus uses, and filters substances such as proteins, viruses, and medications to reduce the fetus's exposure. The placenta begins to form early in the first trimester from cells of the developing embryo and grows in size as the pregnancy progresses. Even though the placenta is delivered and routinely discarded after the umbilical cord is cut, the importance of its proper functioning during the pregnancy cannot be overemphasized.

The placenta is best described as disc shaped, lying against the wall of the uterus. By the end of the pregnancy, the average placenta weighs about a pound, is about ten inches across, and an inch thick. The mother's blood actually leaves the uterine blood vessels to bathe the surface of the placenta, which lies against the uterine wall, before the blood is resorbed back into the maternal veins. This surface is referred to as the uteroplacental interface, and is where the fetus obtains its nutrients from the mother. The umbilical cord routinely comes out of the middle of the other side of the placenta, although in some cases it emerges from near one of the edges. The blood flowing through the placenta is fetal blood—the blood leaves the fetal abdomen through the umbilical cord to enter the placenta, where it gathers nutrients from the maternal blood emerging from blood vessels in the uterine wall, and releases carbon dioxide and other waste products that the fetus does not need. The placental blood then returns to the fetus through the umbilical cord to circulate around the fetus, distributing nutrients and removing waste products of fetal metabolism.

The first sign of a problem with the placenta is usually vaginal bleeding, most often in the third trimester of pregnancy. Any bleeding at this point in the pregnancy needs to be evaluated. This chapter will focus on the placental complications that involve bleeding during pregnancy.

PLACENTAL ABRUPTION

Once the placenta forms early in the pregnancy, it stays attached to the uterine wall until it begins to separate after the baby is delivered. When part or all of the placenta detaches from the uterine wall before delivery, it is referred to as a placental abruption (or abruptio placentae). With this separation, the maternal blood that comes from the uterine blood vessels to interact with the placenta is no longer confined by the placental attachments and is not resorbed back into the maternal circulation (figure 23.1). The degree to which this is a problem relates to how much of the placenta separates and how much maternal blood is lost. Small amounts of separation can be tolerated by the fetus, as the amount of placenta still attached to the uterine wall still provides sufficient nutrient transfer from the mother to the fetus. However, if a large amount of the placenta separates, this may leave too small an area of placenta still attached to provide for the needs of the fetus, and the fetus can deteriorate rapidly. Additionally, separation of a large portion of the placenta can lead to a major loss of blood for the mother.

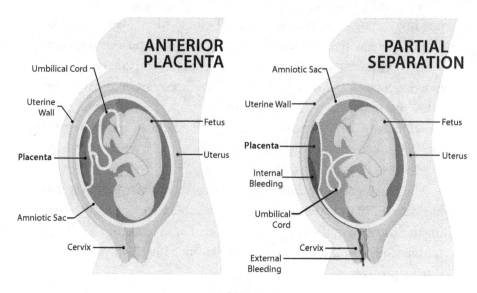
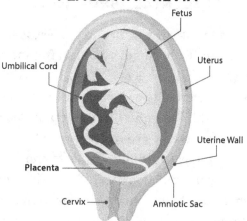

FIGURE 23.1 Uterus with a normal placenta, a placental abruption, and a placenta previa.

Source: Courtesy of Anastasiia Krasavina, iStock.

The most common sign of a placental abruption is the onset of vaginal bleeding at any time during the third trimester. However, not all abruptions result in visible bleeding. If the placenta is located in the upper part of the uterus far from the cervix, the blood no longer being resorbed back into the maternal circulation may not reach the cervix to escape through the vagina. It may collect behind the placenta, which on occasion can be seen by ultrasound. The next most common symptom of abruption is pain over the uterus. This can be either constant or intermittent with contractions, and is not necessarily in proportion to the amount of placenta separating from the uterine wall. Finally, some abruptions are asymptomatic, and only identified by ultrasound or after delivery.

DIAGNOSIS AND MANAGEMENT

If you come to the hospital in the third trimester with vaginal bleeding, it will be important for your care provider to differentiate an abruption from other causes of bleeding including a placenta previa, which will be discussed later in this chapter. Some women can have some bleeding after a pelvic examination or after intercourse, and a speculum exam should be able to differentiate bleeding coming from the surface of the cervix from bleeding coming from inside the uterus. If there is no placenta previa, and no source of bleeding is found from the cervix or vagina, an abruption is very likely. Further assessment will be based on how heavy the bleeding is and how well the baby tolerates it.

If the bleeding is heavy, the first priority is stabilizing the mother and making sure she has not lost too much blood. If the bleeding continues to be heavy and does not stop, cesarean delivery may be necessary to deliver the placenta and stop the bleeding, regardless of the gestational age of the pregnancy and the condition of the fetus. However, bleeding so heavily as to endanger the life of the mother is uncommon. More often the mother can be stabilized, and attention can then be turned to assessment of the fetus. As mentioned previously, larger degrees of placental separation can lead to decreased delivery of oxygen and other nutrients to the fetus. The fetus can tolerate some decrease in oxygen delivery, but if it is prolonged or severe, there will be signs of fetal deterioration on the fetal monitor. Here too, cesarean delivery may be necessary to prevent the fetus from deteriorating further or dying. When an abruption occurs, the stillbirth rate is less than 1%, but abruption accounts for 7% of stillbirths and deaths that occur within a few days of delivery.[1]

If the bleeding is not severe and the fetus is stable, continuation of the pregnancy is likely possible. Continued low-level bleeding is referred to as a chronic abruption. The mother is often hospitalized for a period of time until it appears that she and the fetus are stable or the bleeding stops. Repeat episodes of bleeding often occur, and will still need to be evaluated as above. Further, a chronic abruption may still have some reduction in delivery of nutrients to the fetus, putting it at risk for developing fetal growth restriction.

With the most severe degree of placental abruption, fetal death can occur before the mother reaches the hospital. When this occurs, induction of labor and vaginal delivery may be possible if the mother's condition remains stable, but otherwise a cesarean may still be necessary. If maternal blood loss is excessive, she will likely need a blood transfusion.

Typically, placental abruptions occur in the third trimester. However, there are times when bleeding begins in the second trimester and no other cause of the bleeding is found. This is still likely due to placental separation and is more concerning when it starts long before the fetus has a chance of survival if delivered. Up to 50% of pregnancies with significant second trimester bleeding end with loss of the fetus. The prognosis depends on the amount and duration of bleeding. If the bleeding persists, fetal growth restriction can occur and lead to fetal death prior to reaching the third trimester. Conversely, if the bleeding stops and the fetus continues to grow normally, a good outcome is much more likely.

Placental abruption is more common in patients with hypertension-related complications of pregnancy, and has been observed after blunt trauma to the uterus or cocaine use. It is also more common among smokers. But most cases of placental abruption do not have an identifiable cause, and are not related to any activity or behavior of the mother. When it ends with the loss of the baby it is tragic, but again in most cases it is mild, and a good outcome can be expected. The other good news is that most often it is an isolated event. Although the risk of recurrence in a future pregnancy is somewhat increased, the vast majority of women who experience a placental abruption will have a normal subsequent pregnancy.

PLACENTA PREVIA

Placenta previa occurs when the placenta implants over the cervix (figure 23.1c). This is an uncommon situation, occurring in less than 1% of pregnancies at term, although the frequency appears to be increasing. An ultrasound performed at 20 weeks of gestation will see where the placenta is located, so previas are often identified at this time. However, as the pregnancy progresses the lower part of the uterus elongates, often taking the placenta with it away from the cervix. Consequently, most placentas identified as previas in the second trimester will no longer be previas at the end of the pregnancy.

DIAGNOSIS, EVALUATION, AND MANAGEMENT

There are two main issues with a placenta previa. One issue is that a cesarean delivery will be necessary, as the birth canal is blocked.

Of more concern is the risk of bleeding. As with an abruption, the bleeding risk is mainly in the third trimester, involves the loss of maternal blood, and can vary widely in amount. Indeed, the amount of bleeding can be as little as spotting or a large hemorrhage. If the patient has already had an ultrasound which has identified a placenta previa, it is most likely the cause of the bleeding.

As mentioned above, the lower portion of the uterus elongates in the third trimester, and then the cervix begins to dilate when labor starts. If a previa is present, either of these events can disrupt the attachment of the placenta to the uterine wall, resulting in blood loss. Acute management of the bleeding previa is very similar to the management of abruption. If the bleeding is heavy, the first step is stabilizing the mother. Continued heavy bleeding will require emergency cesarean delivery as the only way to stop the hemorrhaging of the mother. However, this degree of heavy bleeding is uncommon. More often the bleeding will stop on its own, but may recur at any time later in the pregnancy. Once the mother's stability is established, the status of the fetus can be assessed. Different from some situations with abruption, it is most likely that minimal separation of the placenta from the uterine wall has occurred, so that delivery of nutrients to the fetus is routinely maintained. As such, the fetus usually tolerates bleeding from a previa unless it is very heavy. The pregnancy can then continue as long as the bleeding is self-limited, but labor will result in significant bleeding as more of the placenta loses its attachment as the cervix dilates. Repeat episodes of bleeding can occur, and will still need to be evaluated. Cesarean delivery is routinely scheduled for three to four weeks before the due date, at a time when the risks of prematurity are less but before labor is likely to begin. As an example, celebrity Tori Spelling described bleeding very heavily from a placenta previa beginning at 20 weeks' gestation in her fourth pregnancy.[2] She spent the next four months in the hospital with eight additional bleeding episodes, but still managed to deliver at 37 weeks.

PLACENTA ACCRETA

Placenta accreta occurs when the placenta has an abnormally deep attachment to the uterine wall. It used to be a rare phenomenon, but has become much more common over the past few decades. Estimates of its frequency now range from 1 in every 200 to 1,000 deliveries. It is more likely to be present in a patient with a placenta previa and a prior cesarean, so the increase in the incidence of accreta is routinely attributed to the increased rate of cesarean over the same time frame. By itself, it is uncommon for it to cause complications prior to delivery. But after the baby is delivered, the placenta does not release from the uterine wall as it should. Attempts by the physician to separate the entire placenta from the uterine wall are unsuccessful, and only portions of the placenta can be extracted with difficulty. Hemorrhage results, and the only way to stop the hemorrhage is to remove the uterus—a hysterectomy.

TYPES OF PLACENTA ACCRETA

The general term now used for situations of abnormal placental adherence is "placenta accreta spectrum." In this classification system, "accreta" refers to the placenta, which is abnormally adherent to the lining of the uterus. This makes up the majority of cases. When the placenta grows through the lining and deep into the muscular wall of the uterus, it is termed an "increta." In very uncommon situations, the placenta can actually invade all the way through the uterus and into adjoining structures, including the bladder, bowel, or large blood vessels. The deeper the invasion, the greater the risk of major hemorrhage and need for hysterectomy and possible repair of adjacent structures. The overall maternal mortality rate with placenta accreta spectrum is <1%, but it is higher with greater degrees of invasions, and lower in hospitals with a multidisciplinary team and more resources to manage major hemorrhage.[3]

There is also a condition referred to as partial accreta or focal accreta. This is when only a small portion of the placenta is abnormally adherent to the uterine wall. It is only diagnosed at the time of delivery when there is difficulty in extracting the placenta in its entirety. If the placenta is sent for pathologic evaluation, tissue from the uterine wall is identified attached to the placenta, which is not normally seen. There can be increased uterine bleeding with the partial accreta, but most times it can be resolved without the need for hysterectomy. Most patients are able to have more children after this if they so desire, but there is an increased risk of recurrence in future deliveries. Kim Kardashian disclosed that she had a placenta accreta with both of her pregnancies, ultimately resulting in a number of surgeries to repair the uterus but not a hysterectomy.[4]

EVALUATION AND MANAGEMENT OF PLACENTA ACCRETA

Placenta accreta is often first suspected during an ultrasound examination in the second or third trimester. There are certain characteristics of accreta that can be identified to suspect the diagnosis, especially if there is a concurrent placenta previa. Further, the risk of accreta with a previa increases with the number of prior cesarean deliveries, and has been reported to be as high as 60% with three or more prior cesareans.[5] The diagnosis of accreta by ultrasound is usually accurate when performed by physicians with expertise in this area, but on occasion MRI can also be helpful in determining the presence of an accreta and its depth of invasion.

When an accreta is suspected by ultrasound, it should be confirmed by a second ultrasound performed by a specialist with ultrasound expertise. When suspicion remains high, plans should be made for the delivery to occur at a facility with experience with this type of complication. Delivery will require not only surgeons with experience performing hysterectomy and controlling major hemorrhage, but also anesthesiologists prepared to manage major hemorrhage and a well-stocked blood bank. This type of preparation is crucial to reducing the mother's risk of dying from blood loss, and the surgery is best performed under controlled conditions at a scheduled time. For this reason, the recommendation is often made for delivery to be planned for 34 weeks of gestation, to reduce the chances of an unexpected bleeding episode from the placenta previa, and the need for an unscheduled operation. If the mother experiences bleeding prior to this time, she should be evaluated right away so that the appropriate resources can be assembled should delivery need to be performed.

Many patients want more children, and this can be a grave disappointment when a placenta accreta results in a hysterectomy. This has led some experts to attempt to resolve the situation without performing a hysterectomy. After the baby is delivered, the umbilical cord is cut, and no attempt is made to deliver the placenta. If bleeding is not excessive, the uterus is closed with the placenta still inside, and the operation is completed as usually performed. Over the next few weeks the body resorbs the placenta tissue, and any remaining tissue may be removed later by a scope introduced into the uterine cavity through the cervix. Some centers have reported success rates as high as 80% with this conservative approach,[6] with some patients going on to have a successful subsequent pregnancy. Other centers have had much less success with this approach. Leaving the placenta in can result in developing a severe infection or delayed hemorrhage, either of which would require a second operation in the next few days to perform the hysterectomy. The standard approach currently is hysterectomy, with conservative management only considered after thorough counseling about the risks and possible benefits in a patient motivated to retain her fertility.

CASE STUDY #1

Elise was at 20 weeks in her third pregnancy and doing well. Her first two pregnancies were normal, and both were delivered by cesarean at term. At her 20-week ultrasound exam, the fetus appeared to be growing normally, but a placenta previa was identified. Multiple fluid-filled spaces were noted in the placenta, suggestive of placenta accreta. Her physician referred her to a maternal-fetal medicine specialist, who repeated the ultrasound and confirmed that the findings were most consistent with placenta accreta. The risks of this situation were discussed with her and her partner, and plans were made to repeat the ultrasound at 28 and 32 weeks to see whether accreta was still likely. Plans were made for her to have a cesarean delivery at 34 weeks of gestation at a hospital with all necessary resources available.

At 32 weeks and 4 days, Elise began to experience severe abdominal pain over her uterus along with some vaginal bleeding. She was told urgently to go to the hospital, where an evaluation revealed that she was still in pain and bleeding, but both she and the fetus were stable. All necessary personnel were notified, and the blood bank prepared for a multiple-unit blood transfusion. She was taken to the operating room and given general anesthesia. Upon opening the abdomen, blood was noted outside of the uterus, and placental tissue appeared to be coming through a hole in the uterine wall. The vigorous infant was delivered and taken to the neonatal ICU because of prematurity. No attempt was made to remove the placenta, and the ruptured uterus was removed. There continued to be a large amount of bleeding until the hysterectomy was completed, and she was transfused with six units of blood during the operation. Because of the large blood loss, she was taken to the ICU for observation, and then transferred to the regular maternity unit the next day. The remainder of her postoperative re-

covery was normal, but she developed signs of post-traumatic stress disorder from what she perceived as having had a near death experience. She continued in counseling for this for the next six months. The baby was discharged in good condition after a stay in the neonatal ICU of six weeks.

CASE STUDY #2

Willa was at 28 weeks in her second pregnancy when she presented to the hospital with vaginal bleeding. She estimated that she had lost about a half cup of blood, and still had a trickle of bleeding when first examined. Her blood pressure was stable and her red blood cell count was still in the normal range. She was put on the fetal monitor, which showed intermittent contractions, with a normal fetal baseline without decelerations. An ultrasound was performed which showed that the placenta was located on the side of the uterus, not a placenta previa, but there was a blood clot visible just above the cervix. The fetus was normally grown. Willa was admitted for monitoring, but after two days the bleeding had stopped and she was discharged. She presented again to the hospital three weeks later, having passed a similar amount of blood, and the evaluation of both mother and fetus were still reassuring. Again she was discharged when the bleeding stopped, with a diagnosis of chronic abruption.

At 35 weeks Willa now presented with heavier bleeding, and monitoring revealed contractions every four minutes with fetal heart rate decelerations with every contraction. A decision was made to deliver and she was moved to the operating room for an urgent cesarean, performed under spinal anesthesia. A preterm male infant was delivered without difficulty, and the placenta had a clot attached to the maternal side indicative of an abruption of 50% of the placental surface area. Willa did not need a blood transfusion and had a normal postoperative recovery. Her son had mild RDS, which was treated with supplemental oxygen for two days, but was discharged home two weeks later in good condition.

SUMMARY

The placenta is a vital organ of the fetus which is important prior to birth for transferring nutrients to the fetus and waste products to the mother. It normally detaches from the uterine wall after delivery; when it detaches all or in part before delivery it is referred to as an abruption. When this occurs, bleeding can result, which at times can be quite excessive. Bleeding in the third trimester needs to be evaluated to assure the well-being of both the mother and the fetus. If the placenta is located in the lower part of the uterus over the cervix, it is a placenta previa, and can also result in third-trimester bleeding. Diagnosis and evaluation of the cause of bleeding is necessary to direct appropriate management. A more uncommon but very serious situation is a placenta accreta, where the placenta does not detach from the uterine wall after delivery because it had invaded into the uterine muscle. With this situation, bleeding can be excessive and hysterectomy may be necessary to control the hemorrhage.

CHAPTER 24

STILLBIRTH

ONE OF THE MOST DEVASTATING LIFE events a couple can experience is loss of a child. When a baby dies in the uterus during the second half of pregnancy it is referred to as a fetal death or stillbirth. It is sometimes defined as limited to 24 weeks of pregnancy and beyond, but some will also include losses after 20 weeks. Stillbirths occur far more frequently than most people realize, affecting about 1 in every 175 pregnancies.[1] It can happen in a pregnancy with known complications, and it can happen in a pregnancy where everything appears to be going along normally. The only symptom that a mother may notice is an absence of fetal movement at a time when the baby is usually active. When this happens, an ultrasound is performed to see if the heart of the fetus is still beating.

When a fetal death is recognized and confirmed, the health care team needs to provide medical and emotional support to the couple. Some mothers would prefer some time alone with her family first before a conversation is initiated about how to proceed. Once she is ready for the conversation, there should be some discussion as to possible causes, and tests that can be performed to investigate the cause. Assuming that there are no medical complications warranting immediate action, there is no rush to deliver the baby. Some women ask to be able to spend more time with the baby still inside, but most want to move relatively soon to delivery.

CAUSES AND RISK FACTORS FOR STILLBIRTH

The list of complications that can lead to stillbirth is quite long, and includes issues with either the mother or the fetus. Maternal complications which can cause stillbirth include placental abruption, abdominal trauma, seizures, severe maternal infections, poorly controlled diabetes, severe hypertension, elevated bile levels, kidney disease, and substance abuse. Women over age 40 and those with obesity are also at increased risk of fetal death, and it is more common for women with multiple gestations, IVF pregnancies, smoking, and pregnancies that go more than a week past the due date. Fetal conditions which increase the chances of stillbirth include chromosomal and other genetic abnormalities, certain birth defects, intrauterine infections, and fetal growth restriction. There is also a situation known as fetal-maternal hemorrhage, where there is a break in the barrier that separates the fetal circulation and the maternal circulation. When this occurs, fetal blood is lost into the maternal circulation. When the amount of fetal blood lost in this way is large, the resulting fetal anemia can be fatal.

Complications of the umbilical cord have traditionally been thought to be a common cause of stillbirth, and is often assumed when no other cause is identified. However, the cord being wrapped around the baby's neck by itself is very unlikely to be the cause of death. The cord being around the neck is common, being present in about one in four deliveries, and stillbirth is no more common for those situations than when it is not. And since the fetus gets its oxygen and other nutrients via the cord and not by breathing, the cord being around the neck cannot choke the baby. Only if the cord is wrapped so tightly around the neck or limbs that blood flow stops is it likely to cause the baby to die. Other problems with the umbilical cord can be a cause of fetal death, including a tear in one of the cord's blood vessels, a clot or stricture in one of the vessels, or a tight knot in the cord, all of which can interrupt blood flow to the baby.

EVALUATION OF STILLBIRTH

Whenever there is a fetal death, the parents, of course, will want to know why this occurred. When the cause is not obvious from the maternal history and known pregnancy complications, there is a process for the full evaluation, which should be offered to the couple. An autopsy of the delivered baby can identify major birth defects not previously found on ultrasound or examination after birth. Testing can be performed on tissue to look for genetic abnormalities. Pathologic examination of the placenta and umbilical cord can look for clots in major blood vessels, signs of infection, or other abnormalities. And maternal blood should be evaluated to determine whether there is a large amount of fetal blood in the maternal circulation, antiphospholipid antibodies present, or high levels of bile. Some of these tests take days to get a result, with an autopsy often not complete for many weeks.

Even when risk factors such as maternal smoking or IVF conception are present, these cannot be assumed to be the cause of the fetal death. Indeed, up to 50% of stillbirths do not have a definitive cause identified.[2] Most couples find this very disappointing—if no cause can be assigned, how can they be reassured that it won't happen again in a future pregnancy? It should be emphasized that when there is an unexplained fetal death, the recurrence risk for it happening again is very low, at 1–2%. This is a much better prognosis than would be given in the case of stillbirth occurring to a woman with significant kidney disease, or in some other situations where the likely cause is identified.

Emotional support is an essential component of caring for someone who has experienced a stillbirth. Many hospitals have professionals trained in bereavement care and their expertise can be invaluable. But this care needs to be individualized, as patients' needs vary considerably. All caregivers involved should be sensitive to and acknowledge the individual's grief. Assistance can be given in planning for burials or cremation, and making sure the couple is aware of resources available after discharge, including group and individual therapy sessions. Plans should be made as to how the results of the evaluation will be communicated and the implications explained. It should also be recognized that the parents often have feelings of anger or guilt, and it can be very helpful to explain that it is extremely unlikely that the loss was due to anything the mother did or did not do.

Delivery should almost always be vaginal, with cesarean reserved for situations where it is unsafe to wait for the many hours that labor might take, such as if there is heavy bleeding, or in situations where vaginal delivery is not possible, such as placenta previa. If not induced, most women will go into labor naturally within two weeks. But delay in delivery of a stillborn fetus can affect the way a baby may look when it is delivered, and may impair the evaluation of the cause of death. If the baby is small enough, a dilation and curettage (D&C, where the cervix is dilated and instruments are used to remove the baby from the uterus) may be a possibility. This will spare the mother a potentially long labor, but the baby will not come out intact. With some maternal complications, such as preeclampsia, delay may result in a worse maternal outcome. All methods of pain relief available during normal labor should be available for the woman delivering a stillborn fetus.

When a baby is stillborn, the parents may want some time alone with the baby, and they can hold it. They may wish to have family and/or friends there as well, or to have the baby baptized. Many hospitals make footprints or handprints of the stillborn child as a memento, and pictures can be taken. A perinatal grief counselor can be very helpful for the parents to begin the grieving process, and share counseling resources that will be available once they leave the hospital. Some parents may wish to have memorial or funeral services for a lost beloved child. Obtaining counseling prior to or after delivery may help parents weather this very painful storm in a way that is comforting and honors the baby they desired and cherished.

PREGNANCY AFTER STILLBIRTH

Most often, after a stillbirth a woman will want to have another pregnancy. Some will want to begin trying right away, while others may want to wait. There is no accepted time interval as to how long one should wait to conceive again, but three to six months is often recommended. It is to be expected that the mother will be quite anxious throughout the subsequent pregnancy, even if the prognosis for a normal outcome is very good. Patients should feel reassured when they feel the baby moving, and weekly fetal surveillance toward the end of the pregnancy can also be helpful to alleviate anxiety. Mental health counseling and anti-anxiety medications may also be very helpful in getting the mother through this difficult situation. Although delivery before 39 weeks is associated with a small increase in risk of the baby needing some care in the neonatal ICU, many women would be willing to take this risk and relieve some of their anxiety with delivery at 37 weeks, when a pregnancy is considered term.

CASE STUDY #1

Amanda was at 38 weeks in her second pregnancy when she called her physician's office to report not feeling the baby moving for 12 hours. She was instructed to come to the hospital, where an ultrasound was performed showing that the baby's heart was no longer beating. Amanda's first pregnancy had been normal and she delivered vaginally at 40 weeks. This pregnancy had also been normal to this point, and she had normal genetic testing results and a mid-trimester ultrasound showing normal fetal anatomy. Her most recent ultrasound showed normal fetal size and a normal amount of amniotic fluid around the baby. She had no history of diabetes or other medical conditions, and no new issues were identified on this admission. The fetal death was disclosed to Amanda and her partner, who were both quite distraught with the news. After some time alone, it was explained to them that testing was available to try to determine the cause of the fetal death, and they agreed to all tests suggested. Maternal blood was then sent for antiphospholipid antibody testing as well as testing for infections and fetal blood.

When Amanda was ready, an induction of labor was started, and she received epidural anesthesia for pain relief. A perinatal loss counselor met her and a discussion was started regarding her wishes for the baby after it was born. After a five-hour labor, she delivered a stillborn female infant weighing 7 pounds, 4 ounces with no apparent external abnormalities. A chaplain was present for the delivery and the baby was baptized. The placenta and umbilical cord were sent for pathologic evaluation. Amanda and her partner wanted to hold the baby, and they kept her in their room until Amanda was discharged 12 hours later. At this time the baby was sent for an autopsy to be performed. Arrangements were made to communicate the test results to them as well as for a follow-up meeting with the loss counselor.

Amanda and her partner came for a meeting with her physician two weeks later. Preliminary autopsy results found no abnormal internal organs and the placenta was also reported as normal. Genetic testing on fetal blood also showed no abnormalities. She had normal antiphospholipid antibody testing, but there was a large amount of fetal blood found in Amanda's blood sample. This meant that there had been a large fetal-maternal *hemorrhage, and this was most likely the cause of the fetal death. The physician reemphasized that this was not caused by anything Amanda did, and was not preventable. Fetal-maternal hemorrhage has a very low recurrence rate, most likely less than 1%, so the prognosis for a future pregnancy was very good.*

Amanda conceived again four months later. She was reassured by normal genetic tests and a normal mid-trimester ultrasound, and was seen regularly by a mental health counselor with experience treating women who had experienced a pregnancy loss. She perceived fetal movement multiple times a day, and got further reassurance with weekly NSTs beginning at 32 weeks. Induction of labor was scheduled for 37 weeks. She delivered a normal 7-pound, 8-ounce female infant, and both were discharged to home two days later.

CASE STUDY #2

Carly had genetic testing in her first two pregnancies, with cell-free DNA testing showing a low likelihood of a chromosomal abnormality. In her third pregnancy, now at age 39, she again had genetic testing, which now returned with a high likelihood of Down syndrome being present. Carly declined confirmative testing with CVS or amniocentesis, and wanted to continue the pregnancy. At 20 weeks, ultrasound suspected a cardiac anomaly, and a fetal cardiac echo identified tetralogy of Fallot abnormalities, which is more common with Down syndrome. These included a hole between the left and right ventricles, a small pulmonic valve, right ventricle enlargement, and aorta overriding both ventricles. The cardiologist explained that this type of defect would be correctible with open heart surgery.

At 28 weeks, Carly noted the absence of fetal movement upon waking one morning. She went to the hospital, where an ultrasound showed no heartbeat present. It was explained that stillbirth was more common for fetuses with Down syndrome and those with cardiac defects, and the combination of these two risk factors likely explained the loss. Carly underwent labor induction that day, and delivered after seven hours of labor. She declined any further blood tests on her or the baby, and declined an autopsy. A funeral was planned for the child. She did meet with the perinatal grief counselor, and arrangements were made for her to see a therapist two weeks later.

SUMMARY

Stillbirth is a devastating outcome for a pregnancy, and is not a rare occurrence. For women who experience such an event it can be the most traumatic event they have ever had. A thorough evaluation of the circumstances can be very helpful for a couple with this experience, even if no abnormalities can be identified. Fortunately, most often the prognosis for another pregnancy is very good. During a subsequent pregnancy, counseling and reassuring tests can be helpful in dealing with the anxiety, allowing the patient to get to the end of pregnancy and experience a normal outcome.

CHAPTER 25

BLOOD GROUP ISOIMMUNIZATION

BLOOD GROUP ISOIMMUNIZATION is a medical condition that few people are aware of, including most physicians. It mainly affects pregnancy, so it is usually only familiar to obstetricians and blood bank specialists. It happens when the mother's immune system makes antibodies that attach to red blood cells (RBCs) of the fetus and cause them to be destroyed, resulting in fetal anemia. The evaluation process is quite involved, and it is not until you are fairly far along in this evaluation that the seriousness of the situation will be known. If you have isoimmunization it is important for you to understand it, as in some cases it can be severe enough to cause life-threatening anemia for the fetus. Until 40 years ago, this was not a treatable condition, and some women would lose pregnancy after pregnancy. But fortunately, techniques have now been developed so that almost all women with isoimmunization can still have a healthy child. This is but one of several examples where we have made great strides in obstetrics to treat a serious condition.

UNDERSTANDING ISOIMMUNIZATION

Each person's DNA contains genes that code for various proteins on the surface of RBCs, and these proteins determine that person's blood type. There is an A and a B protein—if a person has both A and B, their blood type is AB; if she has neither, the blood type is O. Another protein on the RBC most people are familiar with is Rh, with approximately 15% of people being Rh-negative. If a person is transfused with RBCs that contain a protein that they themselves do not have, the body can recognize it as foreign and will begin to form antibodies against this protein as if it were a foreign bacteria or virus. This will not be a problem unless the body sees this protein again.

Early in pregnancy one of the blood tests routinely performed determines the mother's blood type, and there is also a screening test for her having antibodies against RBC proteins. Since most people have never had a transfusion, the antibody screen is usually negative. If your antibody screen is positive, this could be a problem leading to fetal anemia. For example, if a woman is Rh-negative and develops antibodies against the Rh protein (also known as anti-D), these antibodies can cross into the baby's bloodstream and begin to destroy RBCs if the baby is Rh-positive. There are situations during pregnancy, most often during delivery, where some of the baby's Rh-positive blood can enter the mother's bloodstream. The mother's immune system will recognize the Rh protein as foreign and begin to make antibodies against it. These antibodies do not form right away but can be a problem for future pregnancies. Most situations like this can now be avoided by administering Rhogam to the Rh-negative mother after delivery. Rhogam is actually made of antibodies against the Rh protein, the same antibodies we don't want the mother to form herself. But these antibodies won't attack her RBCs, since she is Rh-negative. The Rhogam antibodies search out any Rh-positive RBCs that might have entered her bloodstream from the fetus or placenta during delivery and destroy them before the mother can mount an antibody response herself. Rhogam is also administered to Rh-negative women after a miscarriage and around 28 weeks in a normal pregnancy, as there are a few cases of fetal blood entering the maternal system after a pregnancy loss and in the last trimester. The routine use of Rhogam for women who are Rh-negative has dramatically reduced the number of women who develop Rh antibodies. Nonetheless, it is still occasionally a problem.

ASSESSMENT AND MANAGEMENT OF A POSITIVE ANTIBODY SCREEN

Assessment of a positive antibody screen can seem quite complicated, but understanding the steps involved will make you better prepared for what comes next. If the antibody screen returns positive, the laboratory will also identify what the antibody is against, and how high the antibody level is in the blood. Some antibodies detected do not cross the placenta and do not cause a problem for the fetus. Others that can be a problem include antibodies against Rh, Kell, Duffy, and some other rarer ones. Quantification will come in the form of a titer, expressed as a ratio. The higher the ratio, the more antibody is present. As an example, 1:64 means there is much more antibody than 1:2. It is rare for an antibody to cause severe anemia in the fetus unless the titer is greater than 1:16, referred to as the critical titer. However, this number may vary in some laboratories.

When the mother's antibody screen is positive for an antibody capable of causing severe anemia, the next step would be to test the blood type of the father. If the mother is Rh-negative, her antibody is against Rh, and the father is also Rh-negative, the fetus will also be Rh-negative and so will not have any Rh-positive RBCs for the antibodies to attack; the antibodies will not harm the fetus. If the father is Rh-positive, he could have either one or two copies of the Rh gene. If he has two copies (homozygous), one will be passed to the fetus, and it will be Rh-positive. If he has only one Rh gene (heterozygous), there is a 50% chance the fetus will get that gene and be Rh-positive, with a 50% chance of being Rh-negative. The good news is that a test has recently been developed that can be done on the mother's blood and tells whether the fetus is Rh-positive, but it is not currently in wide usage. The alternative is an amniocentesis, with the fetal cells obtained tested to determine if the fetus is Rh-positive (see figure 25.1).

If now you are in the situation of having Rh antibodies, an Rh-positive father, and an Rh-positive or unknown fetus, the next step is determined by whether the antibody has reached the critical titer. If it has not, the titer is repeated every 2–4 weeks for the rest of the pregnancy, as it can rise as the pregnancy progresses; as long as it remains below the critical titer, no further action is needed. If it does reach the critical titer, sufficient antibody is present that it can cross the placenta and cause significant anemia in the fetus. But despite a critical titer, many fetuses are able to maintain a sufficient blood count and not be severely anemic. Determination of fetal status used to be done by performing amniocentesis every few weeks, but now it is done using ultrasound. Antibodies do not cross into the fetal circulation in significant quantities until at least 16 weeks, so this testing does not need to begin until the pregnancy is well into the second trimester. The ultrasound focuses on a particular blood vessel in the fetal brain that can be seen reliably, the middle cerebral artery (MCA). Using the Doppler technique on this artery, the velocity of the blood traveling through this vessel is estimated and expressed as multiples of the median (MOM). This Doppler ultrasound is performed weekly for the remainder of the pregnancy to monitor the fetal status. As long as the reading remains below 1.5 MOM, the anemia is stable. When the reading exceeds 1.5 MOM, it indicates that the fetus is likely very anemic and at risk of developing hydrops and then dying if not treated. The fetus needs a transfusion.

What comes next depends on the gestational age. If the fetus is only a few weeks premature, most likely a recommendation will be

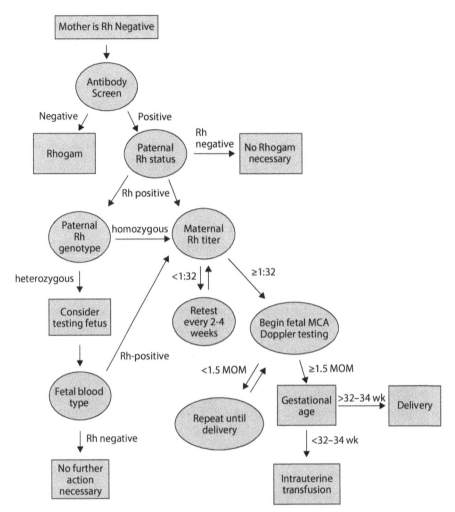

FIGURE 25.1 Evaluation and management of the Rh-negative mother.
Source: Illustration provided by author.

made to deliver the baby and perform the transfusion in the neonatal ICU. Farther from the due date, the risks of prematurity are increased and most likely an intrauterine transfusion will be recommended. This is a complicated procedure with some risk and is usually performed by an MFM physician with significant experience in the procedure. Under ultrasound guidance, a needle is inserted through the mother's abdomen and into the fluid around the fetus similar to an amniocentesis, but the needle is aimed at a segment of the fetal umbilical cord. The needle then is directed into the vein in the umbilical cord, and a small amount of drug is given that paralyzes the fetus for a short period of time. This keeps the fetus from moving around and dislodging the needle before the transfusion is complete. Blood is then transfused into the umbilical vein until a normal RBC level is reached. Even though the fetus is Rh-positive, Rh-negative blood is given so that it will not be attacked by the antibodies that will continue to cross from the mother's circulation.

At this point, fetal blood will be made up of both transfused blood and the fetus's own blood, which will still be susceptible to antibody destruction. Within a few weeks, the remaining fetal blood will be mostly gone, leaving only the transfused blood. Another transfusion will be indicated at this time to again get the blood count to a nonanemic level. Although no further antibody destruction of RBCs should occur, transfused RBCs only last about a month, so further transfusions may be necessary if the pregnancy is still significantly premature. If the severe anemia is found by 20 weeks' gestation, the pregnancy may need as many as five of these intrauterine transfusions prior to delivery.

After the baby is born, it will likely need to be treated in the neonatal ICU. The maternal antibodies that have already crossed into the fetal circulation will continue to attack new Rh-positive RBCs that the newborn makes, so additional transfusions may be necessary. The ongoing destruction of RBCs can result in jaundice, which will need to be treated. However, despite this difficult course of treatment that the mother and then the baby go through, the baby is ultimately likely to do well. These are the babies that would not have survived in the times before improvements in ultrasound technology made intrauterine transfusions possible.

Unfortunately, a patient who has been through this will have similar issues in any future pregnancy. If it is a different father, his blood type should be tested to determine whether the fetus would be at risk. If the fetus is determined to be at risk, maternal titers should again be tested periodically. However, if a critical titer was reached in a prior pregnancy, this step is skipped, and testing should proceed directly to MCA Doppler testing without retesting the titer. All other aspects of management are unchanged.

Up to this point the focus has been on women sensitized against the Rh protein. As mentioned earlier, there are other antibodies that can cause isoimmunization and fetal anemia. If the antibody is known to cross the placenta and cause fetal anemia, it is managed very similarly to management of Rh, starting with testing of the father for the protein. With all proteins other than Rh, it is possible to determine with accuracy whether the father carries one or two genes; thus, it can be determined whether the risk of the fetus being susceptible to the antibody is 50% or 100%. However, there is currently no maternal blood test for fetal blood type as there is for Rh. And there is no treatment like Rhogam to prevent antibody formation to a non-Rh protein. As with Rh, the critical titer is again 1:16. The exception to this is the Kell antibody, where severe anemia can occur at lower titers. If the mother has Kell antibodies and the father is Kell-positive, MCA Dopplers studies are initiated in the second trimester.

CASE STUDY #1

Annika's first pregnancy was uncomplicated, and she received Rhogam after delivery, as she was known to be Rh-negative, antibody screen negative. She had her first prenatal visit in her second pregnancy at nine weeks' gestation, and her antibody screen now returned positive. The antibody was identified to be anti-Rh with a titer of 1:8, suggesting that despite receiving Rhogam she was likely sensitized from the delivery. Testing of her husband showed him to be Rh-positive, so she requested that her blood be tested to determine if the fetus was also Rh-positive. This test result was Rh-positive, so titers were repeated monthly beginning at 16 weeks. At 24 weeks, the titer returned 1:64, so weekly MCA Doppler testing was initiated. The initial value was 1.3 MOM, but by 27 weeks it had risen to 1.6 MOM, and it was decided to proceed with an intrauterine transfusion. When the needle first entered the umbilical vein, a small amount of fetal blood was drawn for testing and the transfusion started. The blood test confirmed that the fetal blood type was O, Rh-positive, and the initial fetal hematocrit was low at 18%, indicating severe anemia (normal is 42-54%). The transfusion was stopped when repeat testing showed the fetal hematocrit now to be 44%. Annika returned the following week for MCA Doppler testing, which was 1.4 MOM, but the week after it had risen to 1.58 MOM. A second transfusion was performed at 29 weeks' gestation, and a third at 33 weeks, when the MCA Doppler reading had risen to 1.55MOM. She was delivered by cesarean at 37 weeks for a vigorous baby girl named Grace. After delivery, the initial newborn hematocrit was 25%, and the baby was transfused in the nursery. Grace required another transfusion on day three and received phototherapy for jaundice. After this she did well without requiring another transfusion and was discharged on day of life 10. Annika was counseled that if she were to get pregnant again, she would begin weekly MCA Doppler testing at 18 weeks' gestation and may again require intrauterine transfusions to achieve a healthy outcome.

CASE STUDY #2

Nina was at 12 weeks when her cell-free DNA test revealed that the fetus was at high risk of having trisomy 18, a chromosomal abnormality associated with multiple congenital anomalies usually incompatible with survival. After confirmation of this abnormality with CVS, she had a termination of pregnancy. She conceived again six months later, but her initial blood tests revealed that her blood type was A-positive with a positive antibody screen. The antibody was identified as anti-Kell with a titer of 1:64, likely sensitized at the time of her termination. Her husband was tested and found to have one gene for Kell, so that the fetus had a 50% chance of developing anemia from the maternal antibodies. Nina miscarried two weeks later.

After counseling about the nature of her isoimmunization and the options for management, Nina and her partner decided to undergo IVF. After successful egg retrieval, 10 embryos fertilized and each was tested for the Kell gene before being frozen. Six of the embryos were Kell-positive and four were Kell-negative. One of the Kell-negative embryos was implanted into Nina's uterus, and pregnancy resulted. The pregnancy progressed normally, and she delivered at 39 weeks a healthy female infant. Two years later, another Kell-negative embryo was implanted and Nina had another healthy girl.

SUMMARY

Isoimmunization is a complex situation that in some cases exposes the fetus to the risk of severe anemia and its consequences. Once the isoimmunization is recognized, there is an orderly process for evaluating the level of risk and the appropriate management. The situation often requires the mother to endure frequent testing, and going through intrauterine transfusions is not easy. However, even with the highest levels of isoimmunization, with the appropriate care that has been developed over the past few years, the outcome for the baby will likely be normal.

CHAPTER 26

CERVICAL INSUFFICIENCY

CERVICAL INSUFFICIENCY (previously referred to as cervical incompetence) is a condition where the mother's cervix begins to dilate in the absence of regular uterine contractions. It is often asymptomatic and occurs in the second trimester of pregnancy. When the cervix opens this early in pregnancy it can lead to infection, rupture of membranes, premature labor, and pregnancy loss. Prior cervix surgery or procedures have been implicated as a cause of cervical insufficiency, but most patients who experience this type of pregnancy loss have no history of cervical trauma or procedures.

Cervical insufficiency is thought to occur in 1 in 200 to 1 in 500 pregnancies. It is not possible to predict who is going to develop this condition. When cervical insufficiency occurs, patients often have symptoms of pelvic pressure, increased vaginal discharge, spotting or bleeding, or contractions. On examination, the cervix is found to be dilated more than is expected by the contractions experienced. Alternatively, when the cervix is noted to be short at the mid-trimester ultrasound scan, cervical examination during a pelvic examination may reveal dilation. Once this dilation occurs, the membrane surrounding the fetus is exposed to the vaginal environment, with its bacteria and acidic pH. Sometimes the membranes will then prolapse through the cervix and extend a significant distance down the vagina. While some patients can remain in this dilated condition for weeks, exposure of the membranes to the vagina can lead to inflammation, which infects or weakens the membranes. This in turn can lead to rupture of the membranes or labor. If this occurs before the gestational age when the fetus can survive outside the uterus, loss of the pregnancy will result. There is also a high risk of recurrence in future pregnancies.

DIAGNOSIS OF CERVICAL INSUFFICIENCY

There are differing opinions in the obstetric community regarding the diagnosis of cervical insufficiency and its management. It is easiest to diagnose when a patient without contractions has a pelvic examination between 20 and 24 weeks and is found to have cervical dilation, prolapsing membranes, and a live fetus in an otherwise normal pregnancy. But the patient is often not seen and examined with these findings because she is not symptomatic. She may not be seen until her water breaks or she is contracting, and it is difficult to tell whether the painless dilation occurred first. When the diagnosis is uncertain, there may be differing thoughts about a plan of management for the current and future pregnancies.

Having a short cervix by ultrasound in the second trimester without a subsequent finding of cervical dilation places a woman at increased risk for later developing preterm labor, but she does not have the above risks related to dilation. Short cervix alone is not cervical insufficiency.

MANAGEMENT OF CERVICAL INSUFFICIENCY

When confronted with a patient with cervical dilation without contractions in the late second trimester, there may be an option of performing an emergency cerclage procedure if dilation is less than

5 cm and sufficient cervical length remains. With this procedure, the patient is given anesthesia (usually a spinal) and a speculum is placed in the vagina. A suture is then inserted through the outer part of the cervix, with subsequent stitches going around the cervix until the first stitch is reached (see figure 26.1). The suture is then pulled tight like a purse being closed, and the suture is tied to hold the cervix closed. Essentially, the cervix is sewn shut for now. If the membranes have descended into the vagina, an attempt can be made to push them back through the cervix before the suture is tied. In this way, the cervix is again closed and the membranes no longer exposed to the vaginal environment.

There are risks with this procedure, and the risks are greater the greater the dilation, the longer the cervix has been dilated, and if the membranes have prolapsed. The needle could puncture the membranes during the procedure, resulting in ruptured membranes,

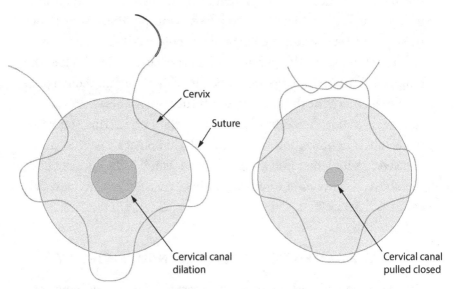

FIGURE 26.1 Dilated cervix with emergency cerclage placement, before and after tying the suture.

Source: Illustration provided by author.

infection could set in, or the patient go into labor anyway. If one of these occurs, it is likely that the pregnancy will deliver soon. Some may argue against the emergency cerclage procedure because the average prolongation of pregnancy from its placement to delivery is 3-4 weeks. But this can be misleading, as most of the losses will occur within a few days, and those patients without a complication in the first week have a good chance of significant pregnancy prolongation, with many making it to term. When the patient does go into labor or reaches 37 weeks, the cerclage suture can then be removed and, when labor does occur, it can then result in a vaginal delivery. It is best to remove the cerclage before labor so that the cervix does not tear.

If a patient had an emergency cerclage placed in the prior pregnancy, or she has a strong history suggesting cervical insufficiency occurring previously, a preventive cerclage is often recommended. This is usually scheduled as an outpatient procedure for the beginning of the second trimester, when the risk of miscarriage has largely passed. The technique is the same as described for the emergency cerclage, but the suture is easier to place and of very little risk because the cervix is longer, firmer, and undilated, and the membranes are not prolapsing.

What has been described above is a cerclage placed vaginally. There are times when a different approach is utilized, placing an *abdominal cerclage*. In this operation done prior to pregnancy or in the late first trimester, the abdomen is entered through a horizontal incision made just above the pubic bone, or using a laparoscope inserted through a small incision just below the navel. A stitch is then placed around the cervix where it meets the body of the uterus. This procedure can be very effective, but is a bigger operation, and the stitch is never removed so that all subsequent deliveries must be done by cesarean. Traditionally, this approach is only used for patients with a prior failed vaginal cerclage, or if the cervix is so short that a vaginal cerclage cannot be placed effectively.

CASE STUDY #1

Sruthy called her doctor's office at 21 weeks in her second pregnancy complaining of spotting and pelvic pressure, and was asked to come to the office for an examination. Her first pregnancy was uncomplicated until 33 weeks, when she was admitted in premature labor and delivered within six hours. When she arrived at the office, she denied painful contractions and leaking fluid. On pelvic examination, her cervix was dilated 3 cm with membranes prolapsing 2 cm into the vagina. She was sent to the hospital and placed on a monitor, and only occasional contractions were noted. A diagnosis of cervical insufficiency was made and Sruthy and her partner agreed to an emergency cerclage attempt after a discussion of the risks and benefits of the procedure. Spinal anesthesia was initiated and repeat examination in the operating room confirmed the findings of cervical dilation without ruptured membranes. After her bladder was filled with a catheter, the membranes receded back into the cervix, allowing a cerclage to be placed around the cervix without puncturing the membranes. The stitch was pulled tight to close the cervix and tied. She was discharged the next day and returned to the office two weeks later, when repeat examination continued to show a closed cervix. She continued to do well, and at 37 weeks the stitch was cut and removed in the office. Two weeks later her water broke and she went into spontaneous labor, delivering a healthy male infant. She was advised that if she were to conceive again, placement of a preventive cerclage at 13 weeks would be recommended.

CASE STUDY #2

Janice was 8 weeks pregnant at her first prenatal visit, where a pelvic examination revealed a cervix less than 1 cm in length. Her prior pregnancy ended at 27 weeks with rupture of membranes and labor after presenting three weeks earlier with rare contractions and cervical dilation of 3 cm. The diagnosis at that time was that she had cervical insufficiency, but cerclage placement was not an option because of minimal cervical length. Given this history, a cerclage was recommended in the subsequent pregnancy, but it was decided that the cervix now had insufficient length to allow for vaginal placement. She was scheduled for abdominal cerclage two weeks later. In the operating room she was given general anesthesia and a laparoscope was inserted into her abdomen through a small incision just below her navel. A suture was placed around the cervix at the place where it met the body of the uterus and tied.

After the cerclage placement, the rest of the pregnancy proceeded without complication. A scheduled cesarean was performed at 39 weeks, and a healthy male infant was delivered. Janice was thrilled that her son would not need a stay in the neonatal ICU and she could take him home with her when she was discharged. She was counseled that the stitch would remain in and would still be effective in any future pregnancy, but again cesarean would be necessary for delivery.

SUMMARY

Cervical insufficiency is a condition where the cervix opens prematurely without regular painful contractions. If it is not recognized and treated in time, labor or infection can set in with pregnancy loss resulting. If it is recognized before significant dilation or rupture of membranes occurs, an emergency cerclage can be placed with pregnancy prolongation, often to term. In subsequent pregnancies, a preventive cerclage can be placed early in the second trimester to avoid a recurrence of early cervical dilation.

CHAPTER 27

MULTIPLE GESTATION

WITH THE MORE FREQUENT use of infertility treatments, the frequency of multiple gestations, including twins, triplets, and higher-order multiples, has now increased to involve 3% of all pregnancies.[1] While most often twin gestations result in two normal healthy infants, risks are significantly increased over pregnancies with one fetus, and this risk is even greater with a triplet and higher-order pregnancies. In addition, mothers with multiple gestation often have more symptoms of nausea and vomiting in the early part of pregnancy, and significant discomfort and limitations in ability to work and be active in the latter part of pregnancy. Twins are termed dichorionic if they have two separate placentas, most often as a result of the fertilization of two different eggs (although some identical twins split from a single fertilized egg and have separate placentas), or monochorionic if they are identical and sharing a single placenta. When a woman finds out that she is carrying more than one fetus, she usually finds this exciting, but she needs to be aware of the risks and extra surveillance and care that the pregnancy will require for both her safety and that of her babies.

RISKS OF MULTIPLE GESTATIONS

The first risk we talk about with multiple gestations is preterm birth. For singleton pregnancies, the average length of pregnancy is 40 weeks, with 37 weeks considered full term; with twins the average length is 36 weeks and with triplets 33 weeks. If twins deliver at 36 weeks, most will do well with a good chance of being discharged from the hospital at the same time as the mother. But half of all twin pregnancies deliver before 36 weeks and 10% deliver before 32 weeks. For triplet gestations, 37% deliver before 32 weeks and 13% at 28 weeks or earlier. Approximately 20% of the babies in a typical neonatal intensive care unit (NICU) will be born as twins or triplets, primarily related to issues of prematurity.[2] As such, babies born as multiple gestations have much higher rates of prolonged hospitalization and serious complications than babies born as singletons. Short-term risks of premature birth include difficulty breathing, bleeding in the brain, bowel injury, serious infections, and vision problems, and these risks are greater the earlier in pregnancy the babies deliver.[3] Childhood issues associated with premature birth include cerebral palsy, lung disease, cognitive impairment, and behavioral issues.[4] Adults who were born prematurely have higher rates of hypertension, diabetes, heart disease, and psychiatric conditions including depression and bipolar disorder.[5] Most of these health concerns occur to persons born at less than 28 weeks. The risks of prematurity are discussed further in chapter 21.

The second risk discussed with regard to multiple gestation is preeclampsia. Women with multiple gestations have two to three times higher rates of preeclampsia than women carrying one baby, and it tends to develop at an earlier gestational age and progresses faster. Mariah Carey[6] and Beyoncé[7] have both spoken publicly about how their twin pregnancies were complicated by preeclampsia, which required premature delivery and long stays in the neonatal ICU before the babies could go home.

The third risk to be discussed is the risk of fetal growth restriction. You can think of this as the ability of the uterus to fully nourish two fetuses being exceeded at some point, so the twins slow their growth to conserve their energy for other essential functions. In fact, the graphs of average fetal weight for singletons and twins begin to diverge at 29 weeks, so that by 32 weeks the average twin weighs about a half pound less than the average singleton. By 36 weeks, the difference is approximately one pound, and this is only true if the twins are sharing the blood supply equally. If they are not, the smaller one will be below the 10th percentile at an earlier gestational age and at risk for deterioration and need for early delivery. Almost 30% of twins will be less than the singleton 10th percentile.[8] These concerns occur at earlier gestational ages for triplets.

The next risk to discuss is postpartum hemorrhage. After the babies are born and the placentas are delivered, the uterus needs to contract down to stop the flow of blood that had been going to the placentas. Because the uterus had been distended further and the uterine surface area covered by the placenta is greater than for singleton pregnancies, contraction of the uterus and cessation of the bleeding tends to take longer and more blood is lost. Medications are available to push the uterus to contract, but these medications do not always work. Fortunately, the mother's blood volume expands more during a multiple gestation, so greater blood losses can be tolerated better. Excessive blood loss is not experienced by most women with multiple gestations. Nonetheless, mothers of multiples are more likely than those carrying one baby to need a blood transfusion. And if the hemorrhage cannot be controlled, a hysterectomy may be necessary to stop the blood loss.

Another risk that is present in identical twins sharing a placenta (monochorionic) is called twin-to-twin transfusion syndrome (TTTS). Monochorionic twins result from the fertilization of a single egg, which then splits into two developing fetuses within the first two weeks after conception. With monochorionic twins there are multiple blood vessels in a single fused placenta that connect the circulations of the two fetuses, so that the blood of one intermixes with the circulation of the other. In 10–15% of monochorionic twins, the amount of blood flowing in either direction is unbalanced so that one of the twins is getting more than its share of the blood volume, and TTTS can evolve. The one having the lesser share of the blood (the donor) will become anemic and have inadequate nutrition, causing the fetus to slow its growth. If this progresses further, the amount of fluid around the baby will decrease, a sign of poor kidney function. The recipient twin will become larger than average, have excess amniotic fluid, and fluid overload in its circulation, which can lead to cardiac dysfunction. If one of the twins dies inside the uterus as a result, it could lead to the death of the remaining twin if left undelivered. Monochorionic twins are also at increased risk of having birth defects, most often cardiac malformations.

MANAGEMENT OF MULTIPLE GESTATION

The first thing in management of twins is to determine whether they are dichorionic with separate placentas or monochorionic and sharing the same placenta. This is best done by ultrasound in the first trimester. TTTS can also be seen in a triplet gestation if two are identical, so determining whether placental sharing is present is important. If it is found, surveillance for TTTS should start by 16 weeks with ultrasound every two weeks looking for size discrepancy between the two and whether the amount of amniotic fluid surrounding each twin is normal. An ultrasound around 20 weeks should look for cardiac defects in each twin, often performed as a fetal cardiac echo. Fetal surveillance at least weekly should be initiated around 32 weeks. For twins not sharing a placenta (dichorionic), ultrasound every month in the second half of the pregnancy may be sufficient to tell whether fetal growth restriction is developing in either twin. If fetal growth restriction is identified, fetal surveillance is begun as described in chapter 18. For all twins, taking a low-dose aspirin, under the advisement of your physician, beginning by the end of the first trimester may reduce the risk of developing preeclampsia. No other interventions, including bed rest, have been shown to be effective in preventing either preeclampsia or preterm birth.

After the finding of a multiple gestation by ultrasound, a discussion needs to be had with your physician about the risks involved and the plan of care. Some women are not willing to accept these risks, most often those with three or more fetuses developing. In this situation, there is an option of "reducing" the pregnancy to a smaller number of fetuses, called selective reduction. Currently it is most often used to reduce triplets to twins, and performed at the end of the first trimester or early second trimester. A needle is inserted into the mother's lower abdomen under ultrasound guidance, and into the sac of one of the fetuses. A toxic medication is injected and then the needle is removed. Some women opt for genetic testing of each fetus with CVS before this procedure, and the reduction then is performed on any fetus found to have a chromosomal abnormality. Selective reduction may also be an option in the second trimester if a fetus is found to have a major anomaly on ultrasound. The other fetus will continue on, and may have less risk than it did as a member of a multiple gestation. Selective reduction is not an option for monochorionic twins.

With regard to delivery, cesarean is usually recommended if the first fetus is not head down. If it is head down, vaginal delivery is usually an option even if the second twin is not head down, though such decisions need to be discussed prior to delivery, and during delivery things can change rapidly and a cesarean still be recommended. Few physicians offer vaginal delivery as an option for women with triplets, but most data show that vaginal delivery is not riskier than cesarean birth for the babies.

If TTTS is identified in identical twins, this is a serious situation with a high risk of losing one or both babies. The most effective intervention if identified before 26 weeks involves a surgical procedure to interrupt the flow of blood between the babies. In the operating room, a scope is introduced into the uterus through the mother's abdomen and vessels that connect the two circulations are identified and interrupted using a laser beam. With this approach, the survival rate for at least one of the twins is reported to be 60–80%, depending on how early in gestation the TTTS occurs and how advanced it is at the time of surgery.

CASE STUDY #1

Tasha came to the office at eight weeks for her first prenatal visit and the ultrasound revealed dichorionic twins. She had nausea and vomiting daily, but this resolved by 10 weeks. The ultrasound at 20 weeks detected no fetal anomalies, but Twin B was at the 20th percentile for estimated weight, with A at the 50th. When the ultrasound was repeated at 26 weeks, Twin A was again at the 50th percentile for growth, but Twin B was now at the 5th percentile, with the amniotic fluid amount appearing normal in both sacs. A long discussion was had with Tasha and her partner, discussing the concerns related to poor growth in Twin B. The size discrepancy was not TTTS but rather insufficient nutrition passing to Twin B through its placenta. This could lead to further deterioration or even stillbirth for Twin B. If it were a singleton, fetal surveillance could be initiated, with delivery performed if the likelihood of fetal death increased significantly. However, with twins, delivery this early for the benefit of Twin B would expose a healthy-appearing Twin A to major risks of prematurity. A decision was made not to deliver for the benefit of Twin B until the risks of prematurity for Twin A decreased, so fetal surveillance for both twins was not initiated until 28 weeks. At that time, Twin A was now at the 40th percentile, and B was now below the 5th percentile, still with normal amniotic fluid volume. Fetal surveillance with weekly biophysical profiles was initiated and was reassuring. However, at 31 weeks, Tasha developed hypertension and new proteinuria consistent with preeclampsia, and she was admitted to the hospital for more frequent monitoring and medication to control her blood pressure. At 32 weeks laboratory tests now showed a decreasing platelet count and a rise in her liver function tests as signs that the preeclampsia was now severe, so a decision was made to move to delivery. A cesarean delivery was performed without complication, with Twin A weighing 4½ pounds, and Twin B weighing 2 pounds, 12 ounces, quite small for gestational age. Tasha was discharged four days later, but both babies had prolonged stays in the neonatal ICU for breathing issues. Ultimately, they were discharged from the ICU and are developing normally.

CASE STUDY #2

Ayala underwent IVF with single-embryo transfer, but an early ultrasound showed two fetuses developing. Repeat ultrasound at 10 weeks confirmed a monochorionic pregnancy. At 16 weeks she began having ultrasound examinations every two weeks, and at 20 weeks her fetal cardiac echo did not find any abnormalities in either baby's heart. However, at 22 weeks a size discrepancy between the twins was first noted, and by 24 weeks Twin A was at the 80th percentile with excess amniotic fluid, and Twin B at the 10th percentile with less than normal fluid. Based on these findings, a diagnosis of TTTS was made. It was discussed that without intervention, both twins would likely deteriorate and die, and delivery would have significant prematurity risks. A recommendation was made for laser surgery to try to separate the blood circulations. The next day, a scope was inserted through Ayala's abdomen and into the uterus under intraoperative ultrasound guidance, and blood vessels connecting the twins were identified. Twenty-two connecting vessels were then laser coagulated and the scope was removed. Follow-up ultrasound the next week showed normal fluid levels surrounding both twins, and by 32 weeks the estimated fetal weight for Twin A was at the 50th percentile and B was now at the 20th percentile. At 35 weeks, Ayala entered spontaneous labor after her membranes ruptured, and the babies delivered soon thereafter. Twin A weighed 5½ pounds and B weighed 4 pounds; both did well in the NICU and were discharged in two weeks.

SUMMARY

Most women carrying twins do well during pregnancy, and have two normal, healthy babies to take home. However, there are significant risks associated with a multiple gestation, with many ending in premature delivery, especially in higher-order multiples (triplets or more). This can be due to spontaneous premature labor, or indicated because of worsening preeclampsia or deterioration of the fetal condition. Monochorionic twins have the additional risk of twin-to-twin transfusion syndrome, but an intrauterine laser procedure may reverse this process and allow the pregnancy to continue further. There are many ways to manage some of the risk factors involved in multiple pregnancies, and you and your medical team will collaborate to address issues as they arise.

CONCLUSION

THIS IS A BOOK about the most common complications that can make a pregnancy high risk. Up to one-third of pregnancies have high-risk issues, and if you have such a pregnancy you are much better off understanding the issues and how they should be assessed and managed. Some of these conditions and complications can be frightening, and the outcome is not always positive. It should be comforting to know that even with some of the most complex situations, very often the results are a healthy mother and healthy newborn. Hopefully, the information in this book has helped you understand the conditions relevant to you, and eased your anxiety.

In planning for a pregnancy with high-risk issues, you should seek out a risk-appropriate care provider. This does not mean that patients with risk factors all need to be seen or cared for by a maternal-fetal medicine specialist. General obstetricians have the experience and knowledge to care for most women with many of these issues. Generalists can care for other issues after consultation with an internist or a maternal-fetal medicine specialist. Midwives routinely care for women with some issues if there is no need to change how a pregnancy is managed. However, there are certain conditions that general obstetricians are not prepared to manage alone, such as isoimmunization described in chapter 25. It must be recognized that MFM specialists are not available in all localities, so patients with complex issues may need to travel to get risk-appropriate care.

In the first two parts, we reviewed issues that can arise before pregnancy and in the first trimester. Preparation for pregnancy may include discussing pregnancy with your primary care provider for any existing medical issues, changing medications to those more appropriate for pregnancy, improving your physical conditioning or losing weight, or stopping smoking. In identifying who will care for you during the pregnancy, you should feel comfortable with their expertise and how they communicate with you. When no longer using birth control, taking a home pregnancy test soon after your period is missed will allow for early recognition of the pregnancy and making an appointment for care. You and your partner also need to consider whether or not you desire to have genetic testing.

Most pregnancies with high-risk issues will have more ultrasound examinations than low-risk pregnancies. Ultrasound is an indispensable tool for diagnosing fetal abnormalities, measuring fetal growth, evaluating fetal well-being, determining the progression of complications, and supporting interventions such as amniocentesis, intrauterine transfusions, and fetal surgery. These are all important medical uses of technology, with no demonstrable risk to the fetus. Most women appreciate the ability to observe the image and movement of the fetus during these exams. You should not be afraid of having too many ultrasound exams if they are judged to be necessary by your physician.

Many of the conditions described in this book are treated with medications. Most of these medications have been used extensively without any significant risks seen, even though their labeling does not say they are safe for use in pregnancy. This is due to the difficulty in doing studies that prove safety of any drug during pregnancy. So even if there is some theoretical risk of a rare complication, you should feel comfortable with medications that have a long track record of use in pregnancy without an increase in complications, as the benefits to be gained outweigh these theoretical concerns. We want to be cautious about medication use during pregnancy to avoid causing harm, but not at the expense of missing the opportunity to improve the pregnancy outcome for both mother and child.

Communication with providers of both your obstetric and medical care is the key to understanding your situation, and how it will be managed. And this understanding will give you more confidence that you are receiving the best care for you and your baby. Choosing a provider with good communication skills is easier today, with online reviews available for virtually everyone in the medical field. Yet it is still best to trust your instincts upon meeting face to face.

Last but definitely not least, attention needs to be paid to your mental health and well-being. Even without complications, pregnancy can be a stressful time, and high-risk issues will definitely create significant anxiety in almost every expectant woman. Given the frequency of anxiety disorders existing in the general population, further stress can make pregnancy very difficult. Fortunately, screening for and recognition of mental health disorders including anxiety and depression are now routine, and doctors are more prepared to refer patients to appropriate mental health professionals. If you develop or already have anxiety or depression, it is important for you to discuss your fears with your care provider, and utilize counseling and even medication to address this important health issue.

There are many organizations that have websites addressing topics covered in this book that may be helpful to you. There are also online forums where you can find stories by women who may have had the same issues that you have. In general, the organizational websites include content that reflects expert consensus. In forums you can hear from women who have experienced similar issues, but the advice they were given may not be authoritative. Here are just a few examples of these websites:

American College of Obstetricians and Gynecologists (ACOG)
https://www.acog.org/womens-health/search#q=high-risk%20pregnancy

American Diabetes Association (ADA)
https://diabetes.org/living-with-diabetes/life-stages/gestational-diabetes/diabetes-and-pregnancy

American Heart Association
Heart.org

Centers for Disease Control and Prevention (CDC)
cdc.gov/pregnancy

High Risk Pregnancy Center
https://hrpregnancy.com/patient-resources/online-resources/

March of Dimes
Marchofdimes.org

Preeclampsia Foundation
https://www.preeclampsia.org/women-and-families

Society for Maternal-Fetal Medicine (SMFM)
https://www.highriskpregnancyinfo.org/

What to Expect
https://community.whattoexpect.com/forums/high-risk-pregnancy.html

Hopefully reading this book will answer many of your questions about your high-risk issues, and will assist in relieving some of the associated stress. It may be unrealistic to think that any book will prevent all of your worrying, and the worrying may not stop even when you are holding a healthy baby in your arms. But getting to the end of the pregnancy with a healthy baby and a healthy mother is everyone's goal, and you are now better prepared for this journey.

GLOSSARY

abruption—Also called abruptio placentae, abruption is when part or all of the placenta becomes detached from the uterine wall while the baby is still in the uterus

ACE inhibitor—Class of medications used for blood pressure control and in treatment of some kidney diseases

amniocentesis—Procedure where a needle is inserted into the mother's abdomen under ultrasound guidance, and fluid from around the baby is withdrawn and sent for testing

angiotensin receptor blockers (ARBs)—Class of medications used for blood pressure control

antibodies—Proteins that are part of the immune system which seek out foreign substances such as bacteria and viruses

anticardiolipin (ACL)—One type of antiphospholipid antibody

anti-nuclear antibodies (ANA)—Antibodies present in patients with lupus and other autoimmune disorders

antiphospholipid antibodies—Antibodies that some people make which can target various membranes in the body. When they cause complications, including blood clots and pregnancy loss, we say they have caused antiphospholipid syndrome (APS)

anti-Xa—Laboratory test used to assess the level of anticoagulation in patients on blood thinners

ascites—Collection of excess fluid in the abdomen

atresia—Absence of a passage through a part of the body

autoantibodies—Proteins the body makes that can attack its own organs

autoimmune disease—A condition where the body's immune system makes antibodies that attack its own tissue or organs

beta blockers—Class of medicines that are used to control blood pressure or heart rate

bicornuate uterus—Type of uterine malformation where there is an indentation in the dome which divides the uterine cavity into two sides

biologic—Class of medications now used frequently to treat autoimmune disorders

biophysical profile (BPP)—Ultrasound test of fetal well-being which examines fetal behavior and activity

bradycardia—Abnormally slow heart rate

calcium channel blockers—Class of medicines that are used to control blood pressure

cardiomyopathy—Disease which weakens the heart muscle, decreasing its ability to pump blood effectively

cell-free DNA testing—Testing of maternal blood for fragments of fetal DNA to look for genetic disorders

cerclage—Procedure where sutures are put in the cervix to prevent it from dilating early

cervical insufficiency—Condition where the cervix dilates prematurely without contractions

chorioamnionitis—Infection of the fetal membranes or amniotic fluid

chromosomal abnormalities—Genetic condition where there are extra or missing parts of a chromosome

CMV—Cytomegalovirus, a virus that can be transmitted from the mother to the fetus, causing many types of birth defects

congenital—A condition which occurs to a baby in the uterus

creatinine—A waste product of digestion of protein and the normal breakdown of muscle tissue, a measure of which serves as an indicator of kidney function

CVS—Chorionic villus sampling, a procedure where portions of the placenta are obtained for genetic analysis

cytokines—Small proteins that act as messengers between cells in the immune system; levels increase with inflammation

deep vein thrombosis—A blood clot that forms in a vein or the lungs

diastole—Second half of a heartbeat cycle where the ventricle fills with blood

dichorionic—Twins with two separate placentas, most often as a result of the fertilization of two different eggs

didelphys uterus—Also known as a double uterus, an anomaly with two separate uterine cavities

DiGeorge syndrome—A genetic disorder caused by a missing piece of chromosome 22, which can result in a heart defect, delayed development, and immune problems

diuretic—A medication which increases the amount of fluid excreted in the urine; often used to treat high blood pressure and heart conditions

dominant genetic disorder—A genetic disorder caused by inheriting an abnormal gene from one parent

Doppler study—A type of ultrasound that looks at blood flow through a blood vessel

echocardiogram—Ultrasound used to evaluate the structure and function of either an adult or fetal heart

echogenic bowel—Ultrasound finding where the fetal bowel appears brighter than normal, which can be associated with an infection or genetic disorder

ejection fraction—Proportion of blood sent from the left ventricle into the aorta with each heartbeat

Factor V Leiden—A genetic mutation that can increase the risk of having a blood clot

fetal-maternal hemorrhage—Leakage of fetal blood into the maternal circulation

Fragile X—A genetic disorder that can result in intellectual disability and behavior and learning challenges

Gaucher disease—A recessive genetic metabolic disorder which can result in an enlarged liver, bone fractures, anemia, and seizures

growth restriction—A slowing of fetal growth below the normal range

HELLP syndrome—Hemolysis, elevated liver enzymes, and low platelets, most often found in patients with preeclampsia

Hemoglobin A1c—A test of blood sugar control used for the diagnosis and management of diabetes

HPL—Human placental lactogen, a hormone produced by the placenta in the second half of pregnancy which causes resistance to insulin

hydrocephalus—Collection of excess fluid in the brain

hydrops, or hydrops fetalis—A condition where an abnormal increase in fluid collects in multiple areas of a baby's body

hyperglycemia—Elevated level of glucose in the blood

hyperthyroidism—Overproduction of thyroid hormone

hypoglycemia—Low level of glucose in the blood

hypothyroidism—Underproduction of thyroid hormone

hysteroscope—Instrument inserted through the cervix to evaluate and operate on the inside of the uterus

IgM and IgG antibodies—Classes of antibodies made by the immune system

low molecular weight heparin—Medication such as Lovenox (generic is enoxaparin) used as a blood thinner to prevent the formation of blood clots

lupus—Autoimmune disorder which can affect multiple organs in the body

lupus anticoagulant—One type of antiphospholipid antibody

macrosomia—Fetal growth greater than the 90th percentile

maternal-fetal medicine—Subspecialty of obstetrics and gynecology with further training in management of pregnancy complications

monochorionic—Type of twin pregnancy where a single fertilized egg splits, resulting in the development of twins sharing a placenta

monosomy—A genetic condition in which a person is missing an entire X chromosome

myoma—Also called a leiomyoma or a fibroid, a benign tumor which grows in the uterus

NIPT—Non-invasive prenatal test, another name for a cell-free DNA genetic test

non-stress test (NST)—A test of fetal well-being using interpretation of the heart rate pattern as seen on a fetal monitor

pericardial effusion—Collection of excess fluid around the heart

placenta accreta—A situation where the placenta invades the uterine muscle, leading to hemorrhage at the time of delivery and need for hysterectomy

placenta previa—A placenta that is implanted over the cervix

pleural effusion—Collection of excess fluid around the lungs

polyhydramnios—Excess fluid around the baby in the amniotic sac

propylthiouracil (PTU)—Medication used for the treatment of hyperthyroidism

proteinuria—Excess protein excretion in the urine, caused by preeclampsia or kidney disease

prothrombin mutation—Genetic mutation that can increase the risk of having a blood clot

pulmonary edema—Fluid in the lungs

pulmonary embolism—A blood clot lodged in an artery of the lungs

pulmonary hypertension—Elevated blood pressure in the blood vessels of the lungs

recessive genetic disorder—A genetic disorder caused by inheriting an abnormal gene from each parent

septate uterus—Uterine anomaly with a thin wall of tissue coming down from the top of the uterus

sequential screening—Also called quad screening, a test for levels of certain hormones and proteins in maternal blood as a predictor of fetal chromosomal abnormalities

shoulder dystocia—A situation during delivery where the baby's head delivers but the shoulders and body are stuck in the birth canal

single-gene genetic defect—A genetic disorder caused by a mutation of a single gene

Sjogren's syndrome—A chronic autoimmune disorder causing dry eyes and mouth, among other symptoms

SS-A and SS-B antibodies—Autoantibodies produced by some patients with lupus or other autoimmune disorders which can damage the heart of the fetus

stenosis—Abnormal narrowing of a passage through a part of the body

SVT—Supraventricular tachycardia, an arrhythmia which can occur in a mother or a fetus where the heart rate is very high

systole—First half of a heartbeat cycle where the ventricle pumps blood into the aorta

tachycardia—Abnormally fast heart rate

Tay-Sachs disease—A single-gene genetic disorder causing severe neurologic problems for a baby

teratoma—Type of tumor which can be benign or malignant

thrombosis—Blood clot in an artery or vein

thyroxine—Hormone produced by the thyroid gland

titer—A ratio used in blood tests to describe the level of antibody present

toxoplasmosis—A parasite that can be transmitted from the mother to the fetus, causing many types of birth defects

trisomy—A genetic condition where there is an entire extra chromosome

TSH (thyroid-stimulating hormone)—A hormone produced by the pituitary gland that stimulates the thyroid gland to produce thyroid hormones

twin-to-twin transfusion syndrome (TTTS)—A situation in monochorionic twins where there is unequal sharing of the blood between the two fetuses

unicornuate uterus—A uterine anomaly where only one side of the uterus is present

VACTERL—An acronym for a syndrome with many abnormalities, affecting some or all of the following: vertebrae, anus, heart (cardiac), trachea, esophagus, kidneys (renal), and limbs

NOTES

CHAPTER 1. HIGH-RISK PREGNANCY BASICS

1. Braun D, Braun E, Chiu V, et al. Trends in neonatal intensive care unit utilization in a large integrated health care system. *JAMA Netw Open* 2020; 3:e205239. PMID: 32556257, DOI: 10.1001/jamanetworkopen.2020.5239

2. Grobman WA, Rice MM, Reddy UM, et al. Labor induction versus expectant management in low-risk nulliparous women. *New Eng J Med* 2018; 379:513–523. DOI: 10.1056/NEJMoa1800566

3. Refuerzo JS. Impact of multiple births on late and moderate prematurity. *Semin Fetal Neonat Med* 2012; 17:143–145. DOI: 10.1016/j.siny.2012.01.012

CHAPTER 2. ISSUES THAT CAN AFFECT PREGNANCY OUTCOMES

1. https://www.cdc.gov/tobacco/campaign/tips/resources/data/cigarette-smoking-in-united-states.html?s_cid=OSH_tips_GL0005&utm_source=google&utm_medium=cpc&utm_campaign=TipsRegular+2021%3BS%3BWL%3BBR%3BIMM%3BDTC%3BCO&utm_content=Smoking+-+Facts_E&utm_term=smoking+facts+and+statistics&gad_source=1&gclid=CjwKCAjw_LOwBhBFEiwAmSEQAaEskaNxbeOonGg2XtU2Ut7vUM48zIAf6F8_Fx9z_rQYmutqbjeL3BoCNAoQAvD_BwE&gclsrc=aw.ds

2. Martin JA, Osterman MJK, Driscoll AK. Declines in cigarette smoking during pregnancy in the United States, 2016–2021. NCHS Data Brief,

no 458. Hyattsville, MD: National Center for Health Statistics. 2023. DOI: https://dx.doi.org/10.15620/cdc:123360

3. www.cdc.gov/ncbddd/fasd/alcohol-use.html#:~:text=There%20is%20no%20known%20safe,exposed%20to%20alcohol%20before%20birth

4. Armstrong EM. Making sense of advice about drinking during pregnancy: does evidence even matter? *J Perinat Educ* 2017; 26(2):65–69. PMID: 30723369

5. https://www.statista.com/statistics/798347/number-of-opioid-overdose-deaths-in-the-us/

6. Wilson MC, Jones CM. Epidemiology of the U.S. opioid crisis: the importance of the vector. *Ann N Y Acad Sci* 2019; 1451(1):130–143. PMID: 31378974

7. https://www.cdc.gov/maternal-infant-health/pregnancy-substance-abuse/index.html#:~:text=From%202010%20to%202017%2C%20the,mortality%2C%20and%20neonatal%20abstinence%20syndrome

8. Committee opinion no. 711: opioid use and opioid use disorder in pregnancy. *Obstet Gynecol* 2017; 130(2):e81–e94. PMID: 28742676

9. https://www.marchofdimes.org/find-support/topics/pregnancy/smoking-during-pregnancy#:~:text=Being%20around%20secondhand%20smoke%20during,Pneumonia

10. Hao H, Yoo SR, Strickland MJ, et al. Effects of air pollution on adverse birth outcomes and pregnancy complications in the U.S. state of Kansas (2000–2015). *Sci Rep* 2023; 13:21476. PMID: 38052850, DOI: 10.1038/s41598-023-48329-5

11. Korten I, Ramsey K, Latzin P. Air pollution during pregnancy and lung development in the child. *Paediatr Respir Rev* 2017; 21:38–46. PMID: 27665510, DOI: 10.1016/j.prrv.2016.08.008

12. Reducing prenatal exposure to toxic environmental agents: ACOG committee opinion, number 832. *Obstet Gynecol* 2021; 138(1):e40–e54. PMID 34259492

13. Reddy UM, Wapner RJ, Rebar RW, Tasca RJ. Infertility, assisted reproductive technology, and adverse pregnancy outcomes: executive summary of a National Institute of Child Health and Human Development workshop. *Obstet Gynecol* 2007; 109:967–77. PMID: 17400861, DOI: 10.1097/01.AOG.0000259316.04136.30

14. Fairbrother N, Janssen P, Antony MM, Tucker E, Young AH. Perinatal anxiety disorder prevalence and incidence. *J Affective Dis* 2016; 200:148–155.
15. Sheen J-J, Wright JD, Goffman D, et al. Maternal age and risk for adverse outcomes. *Am J Obstet Gynecol* 2018; 219:390.e1–15.

CHAPTER 3. INCREASED RISKS IN BLACK WOMEN

1. Centers for Disease Control and Prevention, National Center for Health Statistics. National Vital Statistics System, Fetal Deaths on CDC WONDER Online Database. Data are from the Fetal Death Records 2014–2021, as compiled from data provided by the 57 vital statistics jurisdictions through the Vital Statistics Cooperative Program. Accessed at http://wonder.cdc.gov/fetal-deaths-expanded-current.html
2. Howell EA. Reducing disparities in severe maternal morbidity and mortality. *Clin Obstet Gynecol* 2018; 61:387–399. PMID: 29346121, DOI: 10.1097/GRF. 0000000000000349
3. Davis D-A. Obstetric racism: the racial politics of pregnancy, labor, and birthing. *Med Anthropol* 2019; 38(7):560–573. PMID: 30521376
4. Hobel CJ, Goldstein A, Barrett ES. Psychosocial stress and pregnancy outcome. *Clin Obstet Gynecol* 2008; 51(2):333–348. PMID: 18463464, DOI: 10.1097/GRF.0b013e31816f2709
5. Dole N, Savitz DA, Hertz-Picciotto I, et al. Maternal stress and preterm birth. *Am J Epidemiol* 2003; 157:14-24, PMID: 12505886. DOI: 10.1093/aje/kwf176
6. Riggan KA, Gilbert A, Allyse MA. Acknowledging and addressing allostatic load in pregnancy care. *J Racial Ethn Health Disparities* 2021; 8(1):69–79. PMID: 32383045
7. Committee to Study the Prevention of Low Birthweight; Division of Health Promotion and Disease Prevention; Institute of Medicine. Ensuring access to prenatal care. In *Preventing Low Birthweight*. Washington (DC): National Academies Press, 1985.

CHAPTER 4. PREPARING FOR PREGNANCY AND THE FIRST TRIMESTER

1. https://www.health.state.mn.us/diseases/cy/downsyndrome.html#:~:text=The%20risk%20increases%20with%20the,women%20under%20age%2035%20years

CHAPTER 5. MISCARRIAGE

1. Wilcox AJ, Morken N-H, Weinberg CR, Haberg SE. Role of maternal age and pregnancy history in risk of miscarriage: prospective register based study. *BMJ* 2019; 364:l869. PMID: 30894356, DOI: 10.1136/bmj.l869

CHAPTER 6. HYPERTENSION

1. Centers for Disease Control and Prevention, National Center for Health Statistics. National Vital Statistics System, Natality on CDC WONDER Online Database. Data are from the Natality Records 2007–2022, as compiled from data provided by the 57 vital statistics jurisdictions through the Vital Statistics Cooperative Program. Accessed at http://wonder.cdc.gov/natality-current.html

2. Chronic hypertension in pregnancy. ACOG Practice Bulletin No. 203. American College of Obstetricians and Gynecologists. *Obstet Gynecol* 2019; 133:e26-50. DOI: 10.1097/AOG.0000000000003020

CHAPTER 7. DIABETES

1. Gabbay-Benziv R, Reece EA, Wang F, Yang P. Birth defects in pregestational diabetes: defect range, glycemic threshold and pathogenesis. *World J Diabetes* 2015; 6:481–488. PMID: 25897357, DOI: 10.4239/wjd.v6.i3.481

CHAPTER 8. THYROID DISEASE

1. Lazarus JH, Bestwick JP, Channon S, et al. Antenatal thyroid screening and childhood cognitive function. *N Engl J Med* 2012;366:493-501. PMID: 22316443, DOI: 10.1056/NEJMoa1106104; Casey BM, Thom EA, Peaceman AM, et al. Treatment of subclinical hypothyroidism or hypothyroxinemia in pregnancy. *N Eng J Med* 2017;376:815-825. PMID: 28249134, DOI: 10.1056/NEJMoa1606205.

CHAPTER 10. HEART DISEASE

1. https://www.cdc.gov/heart-defects/data/index.html#:~:text=Heart%20defects%20are%20common,and%20by%20type%20of%20defect
2. cdc.gov/heart-defects/screening/index.html

CHAPTER 11. KIDNEY DISEASE

1. Williams D, Davison J. Chronic kidney disease in pregnancy. *BMJ* 2008; 336(7637):211-215. PMID:18219043. DOI: 10.1136/bmj.39406.652986.BE

CHAPTER 12. BLOOD CLOTS

1. https://www.today.com/health/womens-health/serena-williamss-essay-black-pregnancy-rcna23328
2. ACOG Practice Bulletin No. 196: Thromboembolism in pregnancy. *Obstet Gynecol* 2018; 132:e1–e7. PMID 29939938, DOI: 10.1097/AOG.0000000000002706

CHAPTER 13. UTERINE ANOMALIES AND FIBROIDS

1. Chan YY, Jayaprakasan K, Zamora J, Thornton JG, Raine-Fenning N, Coomarasamy A. The prevalence of congenital uterine anomalies in unselected and high-risk populations: a systematic review. *Hum Reprod Update* 2011; 17:761–771. PMID: 21705770, DOI: 10.1093/humupd/dmr028
2. Wang S, Wang K, Hu Q, Liao H, Wang X, Yu H. Perinatal outcomes of women with Mullerian anomalies. *Arch Gynecol Obstet* 2023; 307:1209–1216. PMID: 35426514, DOI: 10.1007/s00404-022-06557-6
3. Choudhary A, Inamdar SA, Sharma U. Pregnancy with uterine fibroids: obstetric outcome at a tertiary care hospital of central India. *Cureus* 2023; 15:e35513. PMID: 37007410, DOI: 10.7759/cureus.35513

CHAPTER 14. CANCER AND PREGNANCY

1. https://www.cancer.gov/about-cancer/causes-prevention/risk/age
2. Van Calsteren K, Heyns L, De Smet F, et al. Cancer during pregnancy: an analysis of 215 patients emphasizing the obstetrical and neonatal outcomes. *JCO* 2010; 28:683–689. DOI:10.1200/JCO.2009.23.2801
3. https://www.cancer.org/cancer/managing-cancer/making-treatment-decisions/cancer-during-pregnancy.html#:~:text=Chemotherapy%20seems%20to%20have%20limited%20side%20effects,an%20area%20farther%20away%20in%20the%20body
4. Sorosky JI, Sood AK, Buekers TE. The use of chemotherapeutic agents during pregnancy. *Obstet Gynecol Clin North Am* 1997; 24:591–9. PMID: 9266580, DOI: 10.1016/s0889-8545(05)70324-7
5. La Nasa M, Gaughan J, Cardonick E. Incidence of neonatal neutropenia and leukopenia after in utero exposure to chemotherapy for maternal cancer. *Am J Clin Oncol* 2019; 42:351–354. DOI: 10.1097/COC.0000000000000527

6. Cardonick EH, Gringlas MB, Hunter K, Greenspan J. Development of children born to mothers with cancer during pregnancy: comparing in utero chemotherapy-exposed children with nonexposed controls. *Am J Obstet Gynecol* 2015; 212:658.e1-8. PMID 25434835, DOI: 10.1016/j.ajog.2014.11.032

7. Arecco L, Blondeaux E, Bruzzone M, et al. Safety of pregnancy after breast cancer in young women with hormone receptor-positive disease: a systematic review and meta-analysis. *ESMO Open* 2023; 8:102031. UI: 37879234, DOI: 10.1016/j.esmoop.2023.102031

8. Muñoz E, Fernandez I, Martinez M, et al. Oocyte donation outcome after oncological treatment in cancer survivors. *Fertil Steril* 2015; 103:205–213. PMID: 25439848, DOI: 10.1016/jfertnstert.2014.09.027

CHAPTER 15. BIRTH DEFECTS

1. https://www.cdc.gov/birth-defects/index.html#:~:text=About%20one%20in%20every%2033,healthy%20behaviors%20before%20becoming%20pregnant

2. Biggio, JR. Principles of genetics and genomics. In: Norton ME, Kuller JA, Dugoff L, eds. *Perinatal Genetics*. St. Louis, Missouri: Elsevier; 2019:1–10

3. Etemad L, Moshiri M, Moallem SA. Epilepsy drugs and effects on fetal development: potential mechanisms. *J Res Med Sci* 2012; 17:876–881. PMID: 23826017

4. Mother To Baby | Fact Sheets [Internet]. Brentwood (TN): Organization of Teratology Information Specialists (OTIS); 1994–. Isotretinoin (Accutane®) 2023 Oct. Available from: https://www.ncbi.nlm.nih.gov/books/NBK582775/

5. Adzick NS, Thom EA, Spong CY, et al. A randomized trial of prenatal versus postnatal repair of myelmeningocele. *N Engl J Med* 2011. 364:993–1004. PMID: PMC3770179, DOI: 10.1056/NEJMoa1014379

CHAPTER 18. FETAL GROWTH RESTRICTION

1. GRIT Study Group. A randomized trial of timed delivery for the compromised preterm fetus: short term outcomes and Bayesian interpretation. *BJOG* 2003; 110:27–32. PMID: 12504932; Boers KE, Vijgen SMC, Bijlenga D, et al. Induction versus expectant monitoring for intrauterine growth restriction at term: randomized equivalence trial (DIGITAT). *BMJ* 2010; 341:c7087. PMID: 21177352, DOI: 10.1136/bmj.c7087

2. Filipecka-Tyczka D, Jakiel G, Kajdy A, Rabijewski M. Is growth restriction in twin pregnancies a double challenge?—A narrative review. *J Mother Child* 2020; 24:24–30. PMID: 34233387, DOI: 10.34763/jmotherandchild.20202404.d-20-00016

3. Wilk C, Arab S, Czuzoj-Shulman N, Abenhaim HA. Influence of intrauterine growth restriction on caesarean delivery risk among preterm pregnancies undergoing induction of labor for hypertensive disease. *J Obstet Gynaecol Res* 2019; 45:1860–1865. PMID: 31290217, DOI: 10.1111/jog.14062

4. Cho WK, Suh B-K. Catch-up growth and catch-up fat in children born small for gestational age. *Korean J Pediatr* 2016; 59:1–7. PMID: 26893597, DOI: 10.3345/kjp.2016.59.1.1

CHAPTER 19. CONGENITAL INFECTIONS

1. https://www.childrenshospital.org/conditions/toxoplasmosis
2. https://www.statista.com/statistics/626774/number-of-cases-of-syphilis-in-the-us/
3. https://www.cdc.gov/nchs/products/databriefs/db496.htm#:~:text=The%20rate%20of%20maternal%20syphilis%20increased%20222%25%20from%202016%20to,)%20to%202022%20(280.4)
4. https://www.cdc.gov/zika/zika-cases-us/index.html

CHAPTER 21. PRETERM BIRTH

1. Waitzman NJ, Jalali A, Grosse SD. Preterm birth lifetime costs in the United States in 2016: an update. *Semin Perinatol* 2021; 45(3):151390. DOI:10.1016/j.semperi.2021.151390

2. Favara M, Greenspan J, Aghai ZH. (2020). Cerebral palsy and the relationship to prematurity. In: Miller F, Bachrach S, Lennon N, O'Neil ME, eds. *Cerebral Palsy*. Springer, Cham. https://doi.org/10.1007/978-3-319-74558-9_1

3. Janvier A, Spelke B, Barrington KJ. The epidemic of multiple gestations and neonatal intensive care unit use: the cost of irresponsibility. *J Pediatr* 2011; 159:409–13. PMID: 21489562, DOI: 10.1016/j.jpeds.2011.02.017

4. Loftin RW, Habli M, Snyder C, Cormier CM, Lewis DF, DeFranco EA. Late preterm birth. *Rev Obstet Gynecol* 2010; 3:10–19. PMID: 20508778

5. Karnati S, Kollikonda S, Abu-Shaweesh J. Late preterm infants—changing trends and continuing challenges. *Int J Pediatr Adolesc Med* 2020; 7:36–44. PMID: 32373701, DOI: 10.1016/j.ijpam.2020.02.006

6. Janvier, Spelke, Barrington. Epidemic of multiple gestations; Loftin, Habli, Snyder, Cormier, Lewis, DeFranco. Late preterm birth.
7. Field D, Boyle E, Draper E, et al. Towards reducing variations in infant mortality and morbidity: a population-based approach. Southampton (UK): NIHR Journals Library; 2016 Mar. (Programme Grants for Applied Research, No. 4.1.) Chapter 3, The late and moderately preterm birth study. DOI: 10.3310/pgfar04010
8. Barfield W. Public health implications of very preterm birth. *Clin Perinatol* 2018; 45:565–577. PMID: 30144856, DOI: 10.1016/j.clp.2018.05.007
9. Konzett K, Riedl D, Blassnig-Ezeh A, Gang S, Simma B (2024). Outcome in very preterm infants: a population-based study from a regional center in Austria. *Front Pediatr* 12:1336469. DOI: 10.3389/fped.2024.1336469
10. Bell EF, Hintz SR, Hansen NI, et al. Mortality, in-hospital morbidity, care practices, and 2-year outcomes for extremely preterm infants in the US, 2013-2018. *JAMA* 2022; 327:248–263. DOI: 10.1001/jama.2021.23580
11. Konzett, Riedl, Blassnig-Ezeh, Gang, Simma. Outcome in very preterm infants.
12. Walters A, McKinlay C, Middleton P, Harding JE, Crowther CA. Repeat doses of prenatal corticosteroids for women at risk of preterm birth for improving neonatal health outcomes. *Cochrane Database Syst Rev* 2022 Apr 4;4(4):CD003935. PMID: 35377461, DOI: 10.1002/14651858.CD003935.pub5
13. Meis PJ, Klebanoff M, Thom E, et al. National Institute of Child Health and Human Development Maternal-Fetal Medicine Units Network. Prevention of recurrent preterm delivery by 17 alpha-hydroxyprogesterone caproate. *N Engl J Med* 2003 Jun 12;348(24):2379–85. PMID: 12802023, DOI: 10.1056/NEJMoa035140
14. Blackwell SC, Gyamfi-Bannerman C, Biggio JR, et al. 17-OHPC to prevent recurrent preterm birth in singleton gestations (PROLONG Study): a multicenter, international, randomized double-blind trial. *Am J Perinatol* 2020; 37(2):127–136. PMID: 31652479, DOI: 10.1055/s-0039-3400227

CHAPTER 22. PREECLAMPSIA

1. https://blogs.cdc.gov/genomics/2022/10/25/preeclampsia/#:~:text
   =Preeclampsia%20is%20estimated%20to%20occur,leading%20
   causes%20of%20maternal%20morbidity
2. https://www.cdc.gov/media/releases/2022/p0428-pregnancy
   -hypertension.html
3. Bartal MF, Lindheimer MD, Sibai BM. Proteinuria during pregnancy: definition, pathophysiology, methodology, and clinical significance. *Am J Obstet Gynecol* 2022; 226(S2): S819–S834. PMID: 32882208, DOI: 10.1016/j.ajog.2020.08.108
4. Ford N, Cox S, Ko J, Ouyang L, Romero L, Colarusso T, Ferré C, Kroelinger C, Hayes D, & Barfield W. (2022). Hypertensive disorders in pregnancy and mortality at delivery hospitalization—United States, 2017-2019. *Morbidity and Mortality Weekly Report*, 71, 585–591. https://doi.org/10.15585/mmwr.mm7117a1
5. https://www.preeclampsia.org/public/frontend/assets/img/gallery
   /D0900705.pdf; Shahul S, Tung A, Minhaj M, et al. Racial disparities in comorbidities, complications, and maternal and fetal outcomes in women with preeclampsia/eclampsia. *Hypertens Pregnancy* 2015 Nov; 34(4):506–515. PMID: 26636247, DOI: 10.3109/10641955.2015.1090581
6. Aspirin use to prevent preeclampsia and related morbidity and mortality. US Preventive Service Task Force recommendation statement. *JAMA* 2021; 326:1186-1191. DOI: 10.1001/jama.2021.14781
7. https://www.preeclampsia.org/the-news/Healthcare-practices
   /understanding-long-term-effects-of-preeclampsia-and-taking-charge

CHAPTER 23. PLACENTAL ABNORMALITIES

1. Tikkanen M, Luukkaala T, Gissler M, et al. Decreasing perinatal mortality in placental abruption. *Acta Obstet Gynecol Scand* 2013; 92:298–305. DOI: 10.1111/aogs.12030
2. https://www.usatoday.com/story/entertainment/2012/10/10/tori
   -spelling-recalls-dangerous-pregnancy/1624557/
3. Matsuzaki S, Mandelbaum RS, Sangara RN, et al. Trends, characteristics, and outcomes of placenta accreta spectrum: a national study in the United States. *Am J Obstet Gynecol* 2021;225:534.e1–38. PMID:

33894149, DOI: 10.1016/j.ajog.2021.04.233; Obstetric Care Consensus No. 7: Placenta accreta spectrum. American College of Obstetricians and Gynecologists; Society for Maternal-Fetal Medicine. *Obstet Gynecol* 2018; 132:e259–e275. PMID: 30461695, DOI: 10.1097/AOG.0000000000002983

4. https://people.com/parents/kim-kardashian-west-had-tough-birth-due-to-placenta-complications-source/

5. Obstetric Care Consensus No. 7: Placenta accreta spectrum. American College of Obstetricians and Gynecologists.

6. Sentilhes L, Ambroselli C, Kayem G, et al. Maternal outcome after conservative treatment of placenta accreta. *Am J Obstet Gynecol* 2010; 115(3):526–534. PMID: 20177283, DOI: 10.1097/AOG.0b013e3181d066d4

CHAPTER 24. STILLBIRTH

1. https://www.cdc.gov/stillbirth/data-research/index.html#:~:text=Stillbirth%20affects%20about%201%20in,the%20first%20year%20of%20life

2. Stillbirth Collaborative Research Network Writing Group. Causes of death among stillbirths. *JAMA* 2011 Dec 14;306(22):2459–68. PMID: 22166605, DOI: 10.1001/jama.2011.1823

CHAPTER 27. MULTIPLE GESTATION

1. Collins J. Global epidemiology of multiple birth. *Reprod Biomed Online* 2007; 15 Suppl 3:45-52. PMID: 18598609, DOI: 10.1016/s1472-6483(10)62251-1

2. Janvier A, Spelke B, Barrington KJ. The epidemic of multiple gestations and neonatal intensive care unit use: the cost of irresponsibility. *J Pediatr* 2011; 159:409–13. PMID: 21489562, DOI: 10.1016/j.jpeds.2011.02.017

3. Institute of Medicine (US) Committee on Understanding Premature Birth and Assuring Healthy Outcomes; Behrman RE, Butler AS, eds. *Preterm Birth: Causes, Consequences, and Prevention.* Washington (DC): National Academies Press (US); 2007. Chapter 10: Mortality and acute complications in preterm infants.

4. https://www.marchofdimes.org/find-support/topics/birth/long-term-health-effects-preterm-birth

5. Crump C. An overview of adult health outcomes after preterm birth. *Early Hum Dev* 2020; 150: 105187. PMID: 32948365, DOI: 10.1016/j.earlhumdev.2020.105187
6. https://www.hollywoodreporter.com/news/general-news/mariah-carey-nick-cannon-babies-252167/
7. https://www.elle.com/culture/celebrities/a22651522/beyonce-twin-sir-rumi-emergency-birth-post-baby-body/
8. Giorgione V, Briffa C, Di Fabrizio C, Bhate R, Khalil A. Perinatal outcomes of small for gestational age in twin pregnancies: twin vs. singleton charts. *J Clin Med* 2021 Feb 8;10(4):643. PMID: 33567545, DOI: 10.3390/jcm10040643

INDEX

abruption, placental: asymptomatic, 193; definition, 191; diagnosis, 193–95; fibroids and, 104; hypertension-related pregnancy, 195; IVF pregnancy, 15; leading to fetal growth restriction, 144; management of, 193–95; with preeclampsia, 182; and preterm birth, 172; prognosis, 194–95; recurrence, 195; smoking as cause of, 11; symptom of, 193; ultrasound findings, 193; uterus with, 191–92; vaginal bleeding, 193
ACE inhibitors, 47, 48, 88, 91, 92
acetaminophen (Tylenol), 7
adult-onset diabetes. *See* type II diabetes
alcohol use: fetal alcohol syndrome disorders, 12; government warning, 11–12
American Board of Obstetrics and Gynecology (ABOG), 4

American College of Obstetricians and Gynecologists (ACOG), 13, 66, 176
amniocentesis, 31, 32, 216, 235; chromosomal abnormality, 31; for cytomegalovirus (CMV) DNA detection, 154, 160; fetal anemia determination, 214; fetal growth restriction, 150–51; for genetic abnormalities, 120, 130, 131; hydrops fetalis, 167
amniotic fluid, 145, 146, 149–50, 156
anemia, fetal: cause of hydrops, 162–65; cause of stillbirth, 204; cause of tachycardia, 137; due to blood group isoimmunization, 211–17; due to parvovirus, 157; due to syphilis, 156
angiotensin receptor blockers (ARBs), 47
anticardiolipin antibody (ACL), 72
anticoagulation, 81, 95, 98
antinuclear antibodies (ANA), 69

antiphospholipid antibodies, 72, 76, 95, 205. *See also* antiphospholipid antibody syndrome
antiphospholipid antibody syndrome: associated with LAC and ACL, 72; definition, 72; management of, 73; prognosis, 72; severe preeclampsia, 72–73
anti-SS-A antibody, 71, 74, 139–40
anti-SS-B antibody, 71, 74, 76, 77, 139–40
anxiety, 3, 7, 236; alcohol use as cause of, 12; during pregnancy, 16; genetic syndromes, 120; hyperthyroidism as cause of, 63; levels of, 23; medications, 207; sertraline for, 8
aortic valve stenosis, 81
arcuate uterus, 101
ascites, 164
aspirin, low-dose, 18, 47, 58, 73, 183, 230
attention deficit hyperactivity disorder (ADHD), 173
autoimmune disorders, 77; antiphospholipid antibody syndrome, 72–73; azathioprine, 74; biologics, 74–75; case studies, 75–77; Crohn's syndrome, 74; disease control, 70; and fetal bradycardia, 139; rheumatoid arthritis, 74; scleroderma, 74; Sjogren's syndrome, 74, 138; SS-A and SS-B antibodies test, 74; systemic lupus erythematosus, 69. *See also* type I diabetes; systemic lupus erythematosus

betamethasone, 175
bicornuate uterus, 100–101
biophysical profile (BPP): for antiphospholipid syndrome, 73; for diabetes, 56, 59; for fetal growth restriction, 146–47; for hypertension, 45–46; for lupus, 71; maternal age, 18; performance of, 45–46; for preeclampsia, 184
birth defects: alcohol-consumption risk of, 11–12; case studies, 124–26; chemotherapy and, 108–9; clinical consequence, 117; counseling to patient, 122–23, 126; diagnosis of, 122; in different organ systems, 117–19; dominant disorders, 120–21; genetic syndromes, 30, 117, 120; intrauterine surgery for, 123–24; management of, 122–23; maternal diabetes, 51, 54–55, 121; medication associated with, 6, 64, 121; obesity risk of, 21; recessive disorder, 121; risk factors for, 119; seizure medication as cause of, 121; single-gene defect inherited, 120; smoking as cause of, 11; ultrasound examination, 117, 122, 126; VACTERL, 120; viral infections, 121
birth weight, 143, 148
Black women: access to quality health care, 23–24; environmental issues, 21; genetics, 24; implicit and explicit bias, 22; maternal mortality rates, 20, 21; preexisting conditions, 21; psychosocial stress, 23; rate of fetal and neonatal death, 20
blighted ovum, 35, 38
blood clots, 98; case studies, 96–98; deep vein thrombosis, 94–96;

high-risk pregnancy in Black women, 21; pregnant versus nonpregnant women, 93; pulmonary embolism, 93, 94–96; risk factors, 94; strokes caused by, 94; superficial veins, in, 94. *See also* deep vein thrombosis; pulmonary embolism
blood group isoimmunization, 211–19; A and a B protein type, 212; case studies, 217–19; for fetal anemia, 211; positive antibody screen, assessment and management of, 213–17; RBC proteins, 212; Rh-negative mother, evaluation and management of, 213–15; Rhogam administration, 212–13; routine blood tests, 212
blood pressure: abnormal, 43–44; control, 47; elevation, 44, 181; medications, 47, 185; normal, 43; readings, 46. *See also* hypertension
bone marrow, 87
bradycardia, fetal, 71, 136–40
buprenorphine, 13

cancer: case studies, 111–12; diagnosis, 106, 107, 113; fertility after treatment, 110–11; recurrence of, 110; types of, 106
cancer, management of: biopsies and surgery, 107; chemotherapy, 107–8, 113; for patient undergoing treatment, 109–10; radiation therapy, 108–9; termination of pregnancy, 109
carbohydrate-limited diet, 54
cardiac stress test, 86
cell-free DNA testing, 32, 130

Centers for Disease Control and Prevention (CDC), 11, 181
cerclage, 221–25
cervical dilation, 220–22
cervical insufficiency, 225; abdominal cerclage placement, 222–23; asymptomatic, 220; case studies, 224–25; diagnosis of, 221; dilated cervix, 220–21; incidence, 220; management of, 221–23; risk of recurrence, 223; rupture of membranes, 221
chemical pregnancy, 35
chemotherapy, 7, 107–13
chorioamnionitis, 175
chorionic villus sampling (CVS), 31–32, 120, 130–31, 230
chromosomal abnormalities, 127–29, 132; amniocentesis, 31; Down syndrome, 18, 30; fetal growth restriction, 144; fetal hydrops, 163; genetic testing for, 29–31; miscarriage, 36; risk by maternal age, 18, 30–31; spontaneous abortion, 36; stillbirth, 204; at time of conception, 36. *See also* genetic abnormalities
congenital fetal anomaly. *See* birth defects
congenital heart disease (CHD): diagnostic techniques, 79–80; DiGeorge syndrome associated with, 129; family history of, 119; fetal bradycardia, 137–38; hydrops due to, 163; IVF, 15; prevalence, 79; risk factors for, 120–21; types, 79
congenital infections, 160–61; case studies, 159–60; chicken pox, 159;

congenital infections (*cont.*)
coxsackievirus, 159; cytomegalovirus, 152–54; parvovirus B19, 156–58; rubella, 158–59; syphilis, 155–56; toxoplasmosis, 154–55; Zika virus, 158
creatinine levels, 87
cystic fibrosis, 129
cytomegalovirus (CMV), 121; asymptomatic, 153; complications, 153; person to person transmission, 153; preventive measures, 154; symptoms, 152; vertical transmission, 152–53

deep vein thrombosis (DVT): CT scan, 94–95; diagnosis, 94; LMWH, 95, 96; management of, 96; symptoms of leg, 94; ultrasound, 94–95
depression, 7, 8, 236; in adults born prematurely, 227; during pregnancy, 16; genetic syndromes, 120; medication, 16; sertraline for, 8
diabetes, 51–60; blood-sugar control, 51; case studies, 60–62; gestational, 54; history, 52–53; hypothyroidism, 65–66; kidney disease, 88; prevalence, 51; type I and II, 53. *See also* diabetes, obstetrical management of; diabetes, risks associated with; type I diabetes; type II diabetes
diabetes, obstetrical management of: carbohydrate-limited diet, 59; frequent glucose testing, 59; glucose tolerance test, 60; hemoglobin A1c level assessment, 57–58; insulin injections, 59; low-dose aspirin, 58; methods of delivery, 59; oral medication, 59–60; periodic ultrasounds, 58–59; routine medical visits, 59; weight loss and exercise, 60
diabetes, risks associated with: birth defects, 54–55; cesarean delivery, 56; fetal death, 56, 204; fetal macrosomia, 56; preeclampsia, 57, 183; shoulder dystocia, 56
diaphragmatic hernia, 117, 124
diastole, 82
dichorionic twins, 226
didelphys uterus, 101
DiGeorge syndrome, 120, 129
digoxin, 138
diuretics, 47
dominant genetic disorders, 120–21, 129
Doppler study: fetal tachycardia, 137; middle cerebral artery, 164, 165, 217, 218; monitoring fetal status, 214; umbilical cord artery assessment by, 145, 146, 150
Down syndrome, 18, 30–31, 128, 163

echocardiogram: congenital heart disease, 80; fetal, 55, 139, 140; left ventricular dysfunction, 82; maternal, 80
echogenic bowel, 153, 160
eclampsia, 44, 180–81
ejection fraction (EF), 82, 83
endometrium, 99
enoxaparin (Lovenox), 75, 95
environment hazards: affecting Black Americans, 21; air pollution, 14; bacteria and virus exposure, 152; secondhand smoke exposure, 14
estimated fetal weight (EFW), 144–45

Factor V Leiden, 95, 96
family medicine physicians, 4
fetal alcohol syndrome disorders (FASD), 12
fetal cardiac arrhythmias: bradycardia, 137, 138–40; case studies, 140–42; irregular fetal heart rates, 137; tachycardia, 137–38
fetal congenital heart defects: diabetes risk associated with, 55; hydrops fetalis, 163; IVF pregnancies and, 15. *See also* congenital heart disease
fetal death. *See* stillbirth
fetal growth restriction: case studies, 149–51; due to nutrient deficiency, 145–46, 147, 151; fetal surveillance, 89, 146, 148; multiple gestation, 147–48, 228–29; risk factors for, 144; smoking as cause of, 11. *See also* fetal growth restriction, management of
fetal growth restriction, management of: cesarean delivery, 148; Doppler study, 146, 147; genetic abnormalities testing, 145; small for gestational age, 143, 148; ultrasound measurements, 145, 147
fetal hyperthyroidism, 136
fetal-maternal hemorrhage, 204, 208–9
fetal surveillance. *See* biophysical profile; non-stress test
fibroids, uterine: asymptomatic, 99–100, 102; benign muscle tumors, 99; case study, 104; intramural, 102–4; by location, 102, 103; management of, 104; single or multiple, 99, 102; submucosal, 102, 104; subserosal, 102, 103; ultrasound, 102
fifth disease, 156–57
first trimester, genetic testing: cell-free DNA testing, 32; for chromosomal abnormalities, 29–31; Down syndrome, 30–31; gene mutations, 32–33; NIPT, 32; sequential screening, 31–32; serum screening, 31; single-gene abnormalities, 33; for women age 35 and older, 30
first trimester, pregnancy preparation and first prenatal visit: components of, 30; conception estimation, 28–29; due date determination, 29; medical history, 29; physical examination, 29; routine laboratory tests, 29; ultrasound at, 29
Fragile X syndrome, 130–31

Gaucher disease, 128, 166
genetic abnormalities: case studies, 133–34; miscarriage, 36–37, 39; mutation, 127–28; repeat expansion disorders, 129–30; testing for, 130–31; variant, 127–28. *See also* genetic abnormalities, management of; genetic abnormalities, single gene; whole-chromosomal disorders
genetic abnormalities, management of: counseling, 131–32; IVF, 132; mental health challenges, 132–33; pregnancy termination rights, 132; stem cell transplants, 132

genetic abnormalities, single-gene: adult polycystic kidney disease, 129; cystic fibrosis, 129; dwarfism, 129; sickle cell anemia, 129; testing for, 130–31
genetic testing options, 29–33
gestational age, 5–6
gestational diabetes, 54; IVF pregnancies, 15; subclinical hypothyroidism and, 66
gestational hypertension, 180, 181
glucose tolerance test, 60
Grave's disease. *See* hyperthyroidism

heart disease: case studies, 84–86; cause of death, 78; congenital heart disease, 79–80; during pregnancy, 78–84; forms of, 78; left ventricular dysfunction, 82–83; peripartum cardiomyopathy, 83; pulmonary hypertension, 83–84; valvular heart disease, 80–82
HELLP syndrome, 180–82
hemoglobin A1c, 57–58
hemorrhage, with abruption, 191; in Black women, 21; delayed, 199; fetal brain, 172, 175; fetal-maternal, 204, 208–9; hysterectomy, 197, 199, 202; internal, 28; with placenta accreta, 197, 199; with placenta previa, 196; postpartum, 228
hepatitis C, 13
hereditary cardiomyopathy, 82
high-risk pregnancy, 234–36; definition of, 3–4; MFM subspecialist, 4–5, 235; maternal-fetal medicine specialist consultation, 27–28

HIV (human immunodeficiency virus): cytomegalovirus, 152; opioid use, 13
HPL (human placental lactogen), 54
Huntington's disease, 130, 131
hydrocephalus, 153, 160
hydrops fetalis, 162–65; case studies, 165–67; causes of, 162–64, 168; definition, 162; diagnosis of, 164–65; from fetal infections, 153, 155–58; immune, 164, 214; non-immune, 164, 168; treatments for, 165; ultrasound findings, 164, 167
hydroxychloroquine, 70
hypertension, 43–47; in Black women, 21; case studies, 47–50; causes of, 43; chronic, 43, 44, 180–81; genetic factor, 43; gestational, 44, 180, 181; IVF pregnancies, 15; kidney disease, 88; proteinuria with, 181; pulmonary, 83–84; risk factor for fetal growth restriction, 144; risk factor for preeclampsia, 183; risks associated with, 45–46; stillbirth, 204; systolic/diastolic readings, 43–44, 47. *See also* hypertension, management of
hypertension, management of: ACE inhibitors, 47; ARBs, 47; diuretics, 47; fetal growth assessment, 47; labetalol, 47; nifedipine, 47; pre-pregnancy medication, 46
hypertensive disorders of pregnancy (HDP), 180
hyperthyroidism: autoantibodies, 63; causes, 63; diagnosis of, 64; elevated maternal heart rate, 64; fetal thyroid, 65; infertility, 63;

mimic, 64; risk factor, 63; symptoms, 63. *See also* hyperthyroidism, management of
hyperthyroidism, management of: labetalol, 64; methimazole, 64; radioactive iodine, 64; screening for, 67; surgical removal of thyroid gland, 64–65
hypothyroidism: autoantibodies, 63; causes, 63; diagnosis of, 65; infertility, 63; oral thyroxine supplementation, 64, 65–66; subclinical, 66
hysterectomy, 197–99, 228

immune system: complications, 68–75; functioning of, 68; against infection, 160–61
incomplete abortion, 35
intramural fibroids, 102, 103–4
intrauterine growth restriction. *See* fetal growth restriction
in vitro fertilization (IVF) pregnancies, 14–15, 132, 183
isoimmunization. *See* blood group isoimmunization
isotretinoin (Accutane), 121

jaundice, neonatal, 57, 153, 156, 172, 173, 216
juvenile-onset diabetes. *See* type I diabetes

Kell antibody, 217, 219
kidney disease: acute/chronic, 88; asymptomatic, 87; childhood polycystic, 88; immune related, 88. *See also* kidney disease, and pregnancy

kidney disease, and pregnancy: blood creatinine levels, 87, 88–89, 92; case studies, 90–92; kidney function, 87, 88, 92; management of, 89; preterm labor, 88; renal transplantation, 89–90; with single kidney, 90

labetalol (beta blocker), 47, 64
left ventricular dysfunction: echocardiograms, 84; hereditary cardiomyopathy, 82; medications, 82–83
low molecular weight heparin (LMWH), 95, 96
lupus. *See* systemic lupus erythematosus (SLE)
lupus anticoagulant (LAC), 72
lupus nephritis, 88

macrosomia, 51, 55–56, 143
magnesium sulfate, 175, 185
maternal age: advanced, 16–18, 83, 172; chromosomal abnormalities by, 31; Down syndrome risk, 18, 30; mother and fetus complications, 17–18; percentage of births by, 16, 17; preeclampsia risk, 183
maternal-fetal medicine (MFM), 4–5, 215, 235
maternal ketoacidosis, 51
maternal pulmonary hypertension, 84
medical abortion, 38
methadone, 13
methimazole, 64–65
miscarriage: chromosomal analysis, 37; first-trimester, 39; incidence, 34; management of, 37–38; physical and emotional recovery

miscarriage (*cont.*)
    after, 38–39; risk of, 35–36.
    See also miscarriage, causes of;
    miscarriage, definitions of
miscarriage, causes of: diabetes, 51;
    genetic abnormalities, 36–37, 39;
    progesterone deficiency, 37;
    smoking, 11; uterine abnormalities, 37
miscarriage, definitions of, 34–35;
    chemical pregnancy, 35; incomplete abortion, 35; missed abortion, 35; threatened abortion, 35
missed abortion, 35, 38
mitral stenosis, 80–81
monochorionic twins, 226, 228–31
multiple gestation, 226–31; case studies, 231–33; fetal growth restriction, 144, 147, 228, 230; frequency of, 226; IVF pregnancies, in, 15; likelihood of prematurity, 227; postpartum hemorrhage, 228; preeclampsia, 183, 227; preterm birth, 227; twin-to-twin transfusion syndrome, 228–29, 231. *See also* multiple gestation, management of
multiple gestation, management of: cesarean birth, 230; early ultrasound, 229; fetal growth assessment, 229–30; laser procedure, 231; low-dose aspirin, 230
multiples of the median (MOM), 214
myometrium, 99

nausea and vomiting: chemotherapy side effects, 107; diabetes, 58; hypertension, 187; multiple gestations, 226

necrotizing enterocolitis (NEC), 174
neonatal abstinence syndrome (NAS), 13
neonatal intensive care unit (NICU), 5, 173, 227
nifedipine (calcium channel blocker), 47
non-invasive prenatal testing (NIPT), 32
non-stress test (NST): for antiphospholipid antibody syndrome, 73; for diabetes, 56, 59; for growth restriction, 146–147; for hypertension, 45–46; for lupus, 71; for maternal age, 18; for preeclampsia, 184
normal uterus, 99, 100
nurse midwives, 4, 234

obstetric generalists, 4, 5
opioid use disorder (OUD), 12–13

parvovirus B19: asymptomatic, 157; benign infection, 157; complications, 157; Doppler assessment of blood flow, 157–58; IgM and IgG antibodies testing, 157; intrauterine transfusion, 158; mode of transmission, 156; symptoms, 156
pericardial effusion, 164, 167
peripartum cardiomyopathy (PPCM), 83
pituitary gland, 64
placenta: fetal blood, 190–91; formation, 190; function, 190, 202; structure, 190
placenta accreta: definition, 197; evaluation and management of,

198–99; incidence, 197; types of, 197–98
placental abruption: asymptomatic, 193; definition, 191; diagnosis, 193–95; hypertension-related pregnancy, 195; IVF pregnancies, 15; management of, 193–95; prognosis, 194–95; recurrence, 195; smoking as cause, 11; symptom of, 193; ultrasound findings, 193; uterus with, 191–92; vaginal bleeding, 193
placenta previa: cesarean delivery, 195, 196; diagnosis, 195–96; evaluation, 195–96; management of, 196; risk of bleeding, 196; ultrasound findings, 195
plaquenil, 70
pleural effusion, 164, 166, 167
polyhydramnios, 164, 165
postpartum depression (PPD), 8
Prader-Willi syndrome, 128, 129
prednisone, 70, 76
preeclampsia, 180–89; antiphospholipid antibody syndrome, 72–73; case studies, 186–88; causes, 182; characteristics, 180–82; delivery, 188–89; diabetes, 51, 55, 57; diagnosis of, 183–84; fetal growth restriction, 144; fetal surveillance, 89; versus gestation hypertension, 44, 181; HELLP syndrome, 181–82; incidence of, 182–83; low-dose aspirin, 18, 58; management of, 184–85; maternal complications and mortality, 83, 180, 182–83; multiple gestation, 227, 231; preterm birth, 172. *See also* preeclampsia, risk factors for

preeclampsia, risk factors for: kidney disease, 88; maternal age, 17, 18; 183, 188; subclinical hypothyroidism and, 66; systemic lupus erythematosus, 70. *See also* hypertension
premature rupture of membranes (PROM), 171, 174–75, 220
preterm birth: betamethasone, 175; case studies, 176–78; consequences of, 172–74, 227; degree of prematurity, 171; diagnosis of premature labor, 174–75; indomethacin, 175; magnesium sulfate, 175; management of, 175–76; in NICU, 178–79; prevalence, 171; progesterone, 176; rate of, 171; risk factors for, 172; short-term risks of, 227; smoking as cause, 11; use of steroids, 175; uterine anomalies, 101–2, 104
primary pulmonary hypertension, 84
progesterone, 37, 176
propylthiouracil (PTU), 64, 65
proteinuria, 44, 181, 185
prothrombin mutation, 95
pulmonary edema, 182
pulmonary embolism (PE): life threatening, 94; low moleculer weight heparin (LMWH), 95, 96; management of, 96; recurrence, 93; symptoms of, 94; ultrasound, 94–95
pulmonary hypertension, 78, 83–84

recessive genetic disorders, 121, 128, 129, 132
respiratory distress syndrome (RDS), 172
retinoic acid, 6

Rh disease. *See* blood group isoimmunization
rheumatologic diseases. *See* autoimmune disorders
rubella, 158–59

septate uterus, 100, 101
sequential screening, 31–32
Sertraline (Zoloft), 8
shoulder dystocia, 56, 143
sickle cell anemia, 19, 128–29
single-gene abnormalities: adult polycystic kidney disease, 129; cystic fibrosis, 129; dwarfism, 129; sickle cell anemia, 129; testing for, 130–31
Sjogren's syndrome, 74, 138
smoking: cessation, 11; during pregnancy, 10–11; prevalence of, 11; secondhand exposure, 14
spontaneous abortion. *See* miscarriage
SS-A and SS-B antibodies test. *See* anti-SS-A and anti-SS-B antibody
stillbirth, 203–10; at age 40 and above, 18; antiphospholipid antibody syndrome, 72; case studies, 207–10; causes, 204–5; diabetes, 51, 55–56; evaluation of, 205–7; fetal tachycardia, 138; genetic syndromes, 120; hydrops, 162; kidney disease, 88; obesity risk of, 21; opioid use, 13; placental abruption, 194; pregnancy after, 207; radiation as cause of, 108; risk factors for, 204–5; smoking as cause of, 11; symptom, 203. *See also* miscarriage
subclinical hypothyroidism, 66

submucosal fibroids, 102–4
subserosal fibroids, 102, 103
sudden infant death syndrome (SIDS), 11
supraventricular tachycardia (SVT), 136–38
syphilis, 155–56
systemic lupus erythematosus (SLE), 69–71; age factor, 70; ANA blood test, 69; immune-suppressing medication, 70; management of, 71; prednisone, 70; risk in pregnancy, 70–71; symptoms, 69
systole, 82

tachycardia, fetal, 136–38, 63, 165
Tay-Sachs disease, 128, 133
teratoma, 119, 163
thalidomide, 6
threatened abortion, 35
thrombophilias, 95–96
thyroid disease: case studies, 66–67. *See also* hyperthyroidism
thyroid gland, 63
thyroid stimulating hormone (TSH), 64
thyroxine: oral supplementation, 64, 65–66; overproduction of, 64; to regulate metabolism, 63; underproduction of, 64. *See also* hypothyroidism
toxoplasmosis: asymptomatic, 155; blood tests, 155; by parasite, 154; preventive measures, 154; ultrasound findings, 155; vertical transmission, 155
triplet gestation, 227, 229
trisomy, 36, 128
twin gestations, 226

twin-to-twin transfusion syndrome (TTTS), 162–63, 165, 228, 229, 231
type I diabetes, 53, 60, 65, 66, 69, 90
type II diabetes, 53, 60, 143, 144

ultrasound, 8–9; birth defects, 122, 126; congenital heart disease, 79; EFW, 144–45; fetal structure and function assessment, 8–9; first prenatal visit, 29; hydrops fetalis, 164; miscarriage development, 28; multiple gestation, early, 229; placenta accreta, 198; routine clinical practice, 8; short cervix, 221; uterine structural anomalies, 37
unicornuate uterus, 100, 101
uterine anomalies, 6, 99–102; associated with fetal growth restriction, 101–2; bicornuate, 100–101; case study, 105; cause of infertility, 101; didelphys, 101; management of, 102; septate, 100, 101; unicornuate, 100, 101. *See also* miscarriage

uterine fibroids, 99, 102–4
uterine septum, 37, 102
uteroplacental interface, 190

VACTERL (vertebrae, anus, heart [cardiac], trachea, esophagus, kidneys [renal], and limbs), 120
vaginal cancer, 6
valproic acid (Depakote), 121
valvular heart disease, maternal: anticoagulation therapy, 81–82; aortic valve stenosis, 81; mitral stenosis, 80–81; rheumatic fever, 80; schematic representation of heart, 80, 81

warfarin, 7, 82
whole-chromosomal disorders: DiGeorge syndrome, 128–29; Down syndrome, 128; management, 132; Prader-Willi syndrome, 129; testing for, 130; trisomy 13 and 18, 128

Zika virus, 158

Explore other books from HOPKINS PRESS

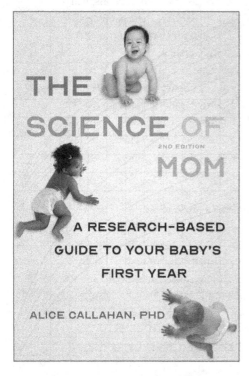

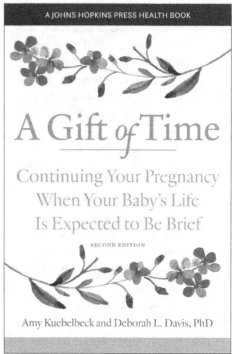

"[Callahan's] compassion and empathy for the difficulties of parenting shine through in every chapter, from breastfeeding to vaccines to feeding to sleeping."

—*Forbes*

"The best resource for parents navigating the difficult journey of baby loss."

— Gina Harris, Chief Executive Officer, Now I Lay Me Down to Sleep

JOHNS HOPKINS UNIVERSITY PRESS | PRESS.JHU.EDU